From Incurable to Incredible

Cancer Survivors Who Beat the Odds

From Incurable to Incredible

Cancer Survivors Who Beat the Odds

Tami Boehmer

Dedication

This book is dedicated to my incredible husband Mike and daughter Chrissy. Thank you for inspiring, encouraging, and supporting me. Without you, I would have never created this book. You're the reason I'm beating the odds every day. I love you.

In Memory

In memory of Jayme Cope, Alan Crace, Marianne Logan, Jennifer O'Neil, Heather Ray, and Anquionette Williams—You bravely faced cancer and will always live on as miracle survivors in my eyes.

And to my dad Irvin Greenfield, stepmother Jean Chesler Greenfield, and grandmother Shirley Reis—I know you would be very proud of this work and how it is helping others.

Acknowledgements

My deepest gratitude goes to all of the amazing people who shared their stories for this book. You are an inspiration to me, and I consider each and every one of you my friend.

I owe so much to my dear friend Jami Elliot, who believed in me and this book enough to generously cover the publishing costs. Your friendship means more to me than you'll ever know. I also want to thank my editor Beth Franks, who patiently guided me through this process far beyond editing copy. I couldn't have done this without you.

Mark and Cathy Lyons, thank you for graciously donating your photography talent to make a middle-aged woman look good. Thanks to Randall Reese, who designed a cover that truly makes the message come to life, and to Ashley Oehler for her keen proofreading skills. And to Jason Bayer, who helped me reach others through his fabulous blog and Web site design.

I want to give a shout-out to Doug Ulman, Lee Boerner, and the rest of the staff at LIVESTRONG, who helped connect me with several of the survivors featured in the following pages. You were extremely gracious with your time and made us feel special when we visited your headquarters. Other people who helped connect me with survivors are: Roberta Hershon from Hope in Bloom, Heather Gregorie, Melissa Drozdowski, Sally DiMuzio, Peter Shankman with Help a Reporter Out, and my personal public relations consultant and husband Mike Boehmer.

To Tracie Metzger and all my other buddies in Pink Ribbon Girls, thanks for your friendship and sending me to conferences to expand my knowledge and meet other survivors. And to all the people who have supported my blog, including Becky Grizovic, Jo Wehage, Dr. Gary Huber, and countless others.

There are so many people in my life who have supported and encouraged me along the way. If I haven't put your names on this page, know that you're always in my heart.

Table of Contents

Part I: Purpose

The author of this book formed her own support group of survivors who beat the odds. By writing about their stories, she helps others and heals her life.

Twice diagnosed with cancer, Greg survived seven surgeries and multiple treatments. He shares what he has learned from his experiences to ease the way for other cancer survivors at the bedside, in the chemo suite, and at his church.

Chapter 3: Erasing the stigma of lung cancer—Deb Violet

When she was first diagnosed, she was afraid to ask for help. Today, Deb boldly pushes for reform to support other lung cancer survivors.

Chapter 4: Living for two—Cathy Wolfe

After she was diagnosed with ovarian cancer, doctors could not guarantee Cathy's survival if she continued her pregnancy. That didn't stop her, and today she has her health, as well as a healthy son to show for it.

Chapter 5: Give strong—Penny Feddick

They told Penny she'd die within a year without a bone marrow transplant. Seven years later, she is still very much alive and is convincing legislators to bring cancer funding to the forefront.

Discussion Questions

Part II: Attitude

Chapter 6: Winning the big game—Bob Kiehsendahl

Bob's game plan for recovery yielded unexpected wins: a lifelong friend and the miraculous birth of a son he was told he could never have.

Chapter 7: Finding the gift in cancer—Brenda Michaels

A victim of childhood abuse who later abused her own body, Brenda used cancer to transform her life. She and her husband now inspire others to find meaning in their lives on their program, *Conscious Talk Radio*.

Chapter 8: Prince for a day—Paul Falk

Paul was nine years old when he was given months to live, but this feisty boy and his mom were ready to fight. Little did they know this experience would later bring them to the nation's capital, where they were given a welcome fit for a dignitary.

Chapter 9: Planting seeds of hope—Ann Fonfa

When Ann was diagnosed with stage IV breast cancer in 1999, she embarked on her own research to finding alternatives to chemotherapy. On September 12, 2001, as smoke billowed from the World Trade Center blocks away, she learned she was cancer-free.

Chapter 10: Cancer is a disease of love—Evan Mattingly

When Evan's mother was dying of cancer, she taught him about the importance of expressing love to the people in your life. Today as Evan faces his own cancer, he heeds his mother's words every day and blesses everyone with his positive outlook and sense of humor.

Discussion Questions   59

Part III: Support

Chapter 11: A mother's love—Rose Paul

Cancer took away Rose's mobility and ability to work, but because of it, she met her soul mate. She credits his love and care for her wonderful life.

Chapter 12: Blessings and blooms— Susan Farmer

Susan had always been a nurturing person, but she found *she* needed nurturing when she was diagnosed with breast cancer. Thanks to a wonderful husband, friends and an organization called Hope in Bloom, Susan was able to recover and give back to others once again.

Chapter 13: With a little help from my friends—Steve Scott

Steve was ready to give up when five different doctors told him he was going to die. His wife, support groups, and friends gave him the gumption to live.

Chapter 14: Hurricanes, humor, and healing—Christine Dittmann

She survived two disasters simultaneously: a dire cancer prognosis and Hurricane Katrina. She keeps her spirit up with writing, parenting, and a little bit of dark humor.

Chapter 15: For the love of Andrew—Patty Mele

Patty always assumed the role of "Super Mom" to her son with special needs. When she was suddenly diagnosed with stage IV breast cancer, she learned she needed to take care of herself before taking care of others.

Chapter 16: Calling all angels—Jonny Imerman

When Jonny was diagnosed in his twenties, he desperately needed to talk to another young testicular survivor. Unable to locate anyone, he founded Imerman Angels, a nonprofit organization that matches survivors worldwide, so no one has to face cancer alone.

Part IV: Perseverance

Chapter 17: Every day is a good day—Dave Massey

Doctors told Dave twice he had six months to live. Now, twenty-three years later, he runs marathons and spreads hope around the country through his non-profit organization.

Chapter 18: A work of art—Yvonne Cooper

After three recurrences, Yvonne discovered a unique treatment protocol unknown to her doctors. Now cancer-free, her colorful and unique ceramic pieces demonstrate her joy, determination, and serenity.

Chapter 19: Riding the distance—Jack Gray

Lance Armstrong was Jack's inspiration for beating the odds, increasing awareness and riding for the cure.

Chapter 20: Hope, faith, and Charlie—Charlie Capodanno

Charlie was just six months old when they discovered he had a rare form of brain and spine cancer. He amazed doctors by his irrepressible determination and remains that way today, nine years later.

Chapter 21: The power of participation—Daniel Levy

The former movie producer launched his own production to unravel the mystery of his diagnosis and find his life-saving treatment.

Chapter 22: Strongest Mary—Mary Jacobson

Before undergoing surgery for a rare form of cancer, Mary bought a coffin and made arrangements for her young daughter. Fifteen years later, she competes in Strong Woman competitions and pulls planes, trains, and automobiles for charity.

Part V: Faith

Chapter 23: Living to serve—Buzz Sheffield

Only God knows why Buzz is still alive more than five years after he was told he had three to six months to live. And that's the point—his faith and service keep him going strong.

Denny asked God to either heal him or "take him home." Thirty-five years later, the answer is apparent.

Kathy felt protected even though she was given little hope from her doctors. Today she shares God's healing message with others through her online ministry.

Doctors gave him less than a six percent chance of surviving, but God had something else in mind. Now Jerry's heeding God's message to him to share his story of healing and hope to others.

Nancy used to be concerned about things like her looks and money. Cancer showed her how to count her blessings for the meaningful things in life.

A word from Bernie Siegel, M.D.

Best-selling author of *Love, Medicine and Miracles; Faith, Hope and Healing*; and dozens of other books

From Incurable to Incredible is a book that everyone should read because it is filled with the wisdom of those who have confronted their mortality and let it become their teacher. When we learn to nourish our lives, we pay attention to our hunger for living. We use it to guide us and heal our lives. Curing our bodies is a side effect.

Self-induced healing is not an accident or a spontaneous lucky occurrence. It takes work, and the work is learning to love ourselves, our lives, and our bodies. When we do that, our bodies do the best they can to keep us alive.

I've learned much as a physician who has counseled cancer patients for many decades. In my latest book *Faith, Hope and Healing*, which features inspiring lessons from people living with cancer, I reflect upon what each story teaches us about not just surviving, but thriving.

I am concerned that readers of this book may miss some of the wisdom it contains because of how simply it is presented by those living the message. In other words, *tourists* often are not aware of what is obvious to the *natives*. So please read the stories slowly and thoughtfully and refer to the common themes addressed at the beginning of this book. These commonalities, coupled with the stories, speak volumes of their effectiveness.

I would also recommend *From Incurable to Incredible* to those of you who are not threatened by illness, so you can live a longer, healthier, and happier life. Remember life is uncertain, so do what makes you happy and eat dessert first.

The Power of Hope

Foreword by Doug Ulman, President and Chief Executive Officer,
Lance Armstrong Foundation

The importance of survivors sharing their experiences is something we stress frequently at the Lance Armstrong Foundation (LAF). When people ask about advocacy and volunteering, I tell them, "If all you do is share your story, you are doing a great deal. It is such a powerful testimony."

This sounds like a simple way to get involved, but its significance can't be measured. Sharing your experience is almost always therapeutic for you, and the benefits to others are far-ranging. That's why stories like those in *From Incurable to Incredible* are so vital. Knowing others have been down the same road is very powerful.

Lance often tells the story of how one doctor said to him, "I like your chances." He said all he needed was that confidence, someone who believed. People want to be inspired and hopeful.

That's why I don't often see the value of statistics. It might be helpful if a doctor told patients that people with this diagnosis have a 90 percent chance of surviving. But telling them they have a 20 percent chance? What does that do but demoralize them? Could you make a statement about the gravity of the situation and still offer hope? I think so.

Hope was something I was certainly seeking when I was diagnosed with chondrosarcoma, a very rare cancer that appears on cartilage. I was nineteen at the time, entering my sophomore year at Brown University, and had no symptoms at all. I went to the doctor not because of any pain, but because of some asthmatic episodes. X-rays showed a shadow behind my heart. We thought it was a heart condition. The next day, I got a CT scan, which showed a tumor they thought was growing for a long time.

It was so overwhelming; I couldn't process it at first. I was shocked, angry, and frustrated. But I went through treatment, and my doctors pronounced I was in remission.

About seven months later, I noticed a mole. I didn't think twice about it, but I went to my dermatologist for a checkup. I was in my dorm room one night when I got a call from my doctor, who said I had melanoma.

This was one of the most devastating days of my life. I had been feeling really good. I had recuperated and gone back to school. Then all of a sudden, I had melanoma, which was another thing I didn't know anything about. Immediately I went through fear, denial, frustration, and anger. My emotions were like a roller coaster.

Three months later, I was diagnosed again. This time, it was a tiny mole—no discoloration or abnormal borders. I just mentioned to my doctor that it was itchy. She said, "With your history, let's check it." They took it off, and said it was melanoma again.

I was very lucky to have an amazing family, great friends, and a network of supportive people around me. My family is really tight-knit and this experience brought us even closer. But even when you have great friends and family, there are times they don't know what to say or how to act. It's not their fault; it's just not what they're used to.

It helped that I'm an optimist. I just approached cancer with the notion that I could overcome this and do great things. There were periods of depression and frustration. But you just hit a point when you stop asking, "why me?" and start considering your next steps. A lot of people around me were very positive and encouraging, and they made a big difference in my life.

It's surreal when you have your whole life ahead of you, and then you're told you have cancer. One of the hardest things facing young people with cancer is the loss of autonomy. As a young adult, you're supposed to become independent. You go away to school or work or are starting your own family. Cancer forces you to be totally dependent on so many people in so many ways, whether it's medical professionals or family and friends, which is a really hard thing to experience.

I was looking for people who understood how I was feeling, but I had trouble finding young adult support groups. Some contacts at organizations even told me young people don't get cancer. That was shocking and unacceptable.

My family fostered the idea that if something is missing in your life and community, you should fill the void and not wait for someone else to do it. So I called my parents and said we should take the lead and start an organization. That was the beginning of the Ulman Cancer Fund for Young Adults, which provides support and advocacy for young adults with cancer.

Right after that, people started coming out of the woodwork and contacting us. They said they felt the same way—they wanted to talk to other young people and couldn't find anybody.

During this time, Lance Armstrong and I first crossed paths. I was playing on Brown's soccer team, which was ranked second in the country, so there were a lot of articles written about my story. A European journalist, who went to Brown and was covering cycling for *The International Herald Tribune,* sent an article about me to Lance.

One day I received an email from Lance. I really didn't know who he was, though I'd heard about a cyclist who had cancer. At the end of the letter he said, "We are the lucky ones. Let's try to find a way to work together and try and change the world." After about three years of emailing back and forth, I traveled to Austin to meet Lance. Shortly after that, he asked me to work with him at the LAF to help young adult survivors. I joined the LAF in 2001 and have been with the organization since.

I'm most proud of the way the LAF is focused on helping survivors. Sure, we're about fighting cancer, but we're also about supporting people and changing their lives. If nothing else, we continue to reach, empower, and inspire them to mobilize. I think people around the globe want to get involved in something that can positively impact others and change the world. At the LAF we're giving individuals the opportunity to do that.

We've funded many great programs and research and have done a lot to get cancer on the agenda, but we've barely begun. I think the millions of people diagnosed with cancer each year deserve an organization that's fully committed to doing everything possible to ensure people won't have to suffer from cancer in the future.

On a personal level, I always look at the gifts cancer brings. For me, one of these gifts was the opportunity to participate, after graduating from Brown, in a hundred-mile marathon in the Himalayan Mountains. It was sponsored by World Team Sports, an organization that joins disabled individuals with able-bodied people to raise awareness of athletes who have overcome adversity.

We ran seventeen to twenty-three miles per day, camping along the way. It was a real physical challenge, but it was also a spiritual and emotional challenge and a turning point in my life. I did something I never thought was possible and pushed my body to a point where I could really trust it again. This felt like a testament to the human spirit and all the people who helped me along the way.

I remember crossing the finish line in a small town in India with people cheering. I thought, "I'm really alive. I'm back!" If I hadn't had cancer, I probably wouldn't have been able to do it.

Another gift of cancer was that I had to mature a lot faster than most people. Now I'm thirty-two and have learned a lot in a short period of time. These are things you can't teach somebody; the kind of lessons that most people learn much later in life or not at all.

None of us know how much longer we have. Life is so short; you have to do what you like. I don't spend much time doing things I'm not really interested in doing. I think we only have one chance here, and I want to make every minute count. I cram as much as I can into every day.

The individuals featured in this book are living testaments to the concept of making every day count. Their stories show that numbers do not tell the whole story when it comes to cancer survivorship. To me, statistics are meaningless. They are based on a whole bunch of people who aren't me. It's impossible to know for certain what is to come.

We do know there is hope, no matter what statistics indicate. For those of us who have been down this path, there is nothing more powerful.

Lance Armstrong Foundation: www.livestrong.org
Ulman Cancer Fund for Young Adults: www.ulmancancerfund.org
World Team Sports: www.worldteamsports.org

Common attributes of "miracle survivors"

A note from the author

When I started interviewing individuals for *From Incurable to Incredible*, I was searching for answers. It was an extremely personal journey. As someone facing a stage IV breast cancer diagnosis, you could say my life depended on it.

My biggest question was: What sets people apart who beat the odds of a terminal or incurable prognosis? As I was putting the stories together, I noticed many similarities among survivors who share their stories. Rather than passively accepting their circumstances; they decided to transform them by:

- Refusing to buy into statistics and the death sentences many of them were given.

- Never giving up, no matter what. They may have had down times, but were able to pull themselves together and do what they needed to do.

- Relying on support from family, loved ones, or support groups. These connections gave them a reason to carry on.

- Choosing to look on the bright side and see the gifts cancer brings.

- Giving back and making a difference in other people's lives, whether it was fundraising, lobbying, or supporting other survivors.

- Having a strong sense of faith. Even if they didn't believe in God, they believed in something larger than themselves.

- Being proactive participants in their health care.

- Viewing their lives as transformed by their experience.

Because they have so much in common, I have singled out attributes they described as being vital to their healing and divided this book into five sections: *Purpose, Attitude, Support, Perseverance,* and *Faith.* To help you get the most of the book and for use in book study and discussion groups, there are questions to consider at the end of each section. Even so, it's difficult to single out just one thing that contributed to these survivors' healing, so you'll notice common themes repeated among the stories.

While I call the individuals in this book, "miracle survivors," overcoming the odds wasn't something that just happened to them. Each person took a very active role in overcoming their challenges, whether it was activating their faith or transforming their lifestyle.

If you find yourself relating to individuals in the book, you're on the right track to healing, health, and joy in your life. I hope reading these stories helps you as much as it has helped me.

Hugs and Healing!

Tami Boehmer

Part 1

Purpose

CHAPTER 1

My story

Tami Boehmer

Age 46
Stage IV breast cancer
Diagnosed 2002 and 2008
Cincinnati, Ohio

For someone who has received a cancer diagnosis—especially a less than optimistic one—hearing an inspiring survivor story is like spotting a rescue ship when you are drowning in a stormy sea.

On February 4, 2008, I was desperate for such stories. Staring at my breast surgeon's forlorn face, I knew something was terribly wrong.

I'd insisted on seeing her a month earlier than my regular checkup because of a large lump I discovered in my right armpit. I had worried from time to time about some swelling and hardness. Since the swelling would go down, my surgeon thought it was probably hormonal. I was so relieved, I didn't question it.

Now I wanted answers. She ordered an ultrasound to determine if it was a solid tumor.

"What do you think it is?" I asked, fear welling up inside of me.

"I think it's a recurrence," she replied. "But we need to do a biopsy to be sure."

"Well, at least it hasn't spread," I said, grasping for any shred of hope she could throw my way.

She looked at me with an expression that I interpreted as extreme pity and remorse. My world as I knew it ceased to exist.

The biopsy results showed it was indeed cancer. The tumor was nine centimeters in diameter, and nine out of fifteen lymph nodes tested were positive. Subsequent CT and PET scans reported that it had spread to lymph nodes in my chest and to my liver.

We decided to go to M.D. Anderson Cancer Center in Houston, Texas, for a second opinion. I figured it was the one of the best cancer centers in the nation; maybe they would have some miracle treatment my local oncologist couldn't provide. They didn't.

At the end of our consultation with the oncologist there, I asked about my prognosis. Suddenly, she scooted her chair up so she was directly facing my husband Mike and me.

"You could live two years or twenty years, but you will die of breast cancer," she said sadly.

In my mind, I was screwed. I knew of several women who died quickly after their cancer had spread. I felt devastated—and angry. I wondered why it wasn't caught sooner.

My first thought was Chrissy, my eight-year-old daughter. I had to do something to make sure I'd be there for her.

During that holiday season just two months before, I shared with a coworker how grateful and happy I was. I had just celebrated my five-year, cancer-free anniversary; I was feeling more competent on my new job, and I adored Chrissy and Mike. It seemed that I could finally push aside my worries and get on with life.

When I was first diagnosed with breast cancer in 2002 at age thirty-eight, my oncologist told me my prognosis was excellent. I had no lymph node involvement. After going through a lumpectomy, aggressive chemotherapy, and radiation, I was declared cancer-free.

Looking at the grim statistics of a stage IV diagnosis, I longed for such rosy optimism. If I couldn't get it from medical professionals, I was going to seek it from others. I needed to talk with other cancer survivors who didn't accept doctors' predictions—people who beat the odds. I was determined to find out how they did it so I could do it, too.

The first person I thought of was Buzz Sheffield, a volunteer prayer chaplain at our church. Buzz always sat in the front row with a snazzy suit and dazzling smile. You could almost see the light of God emanating from him.

The previous year, I had seen Buzz sitting in the courtyard of the large teaching hospital where I worked. It was a beautiful sunny day, and Buzz looked peaceful as he read a book. As usual, I was in a rush. An ambitious public relations specialist, I was dashing to meet a TV reporter who was doing a story on one of our patients.

"What are you doing here, Buzz?" I asked after we exchanged hellos.

"I'm waiting for tests," he said.

"Well I hope they turn out okay," I said, ready to move on to my meeting with the reporter.

"Oh, I have a feeling I know what they're going to say," he said matter-of-factly. "I have cancer all over my body."

I stood there in shock. I never would have guessed that this active, robust man had anything wrong with him. We didn't know each other well at the time, but I felt a special connection with him from that moment on.

After church that Sunday, I asked him about the tests and his illness. He told me he had carcinoid cancer, a rare, slow-moving disease that often attacks the intestines and other parts of the body where hormones are produced. Four years earlier, doctors told him he had only three to six months to live. His cancer was so extensive, chemotherapy wasn't an option. He refused to listen to their doomsday predictions and chose to focus on healing through prayer, giving back to others, healthy nutrition, and exercise. Looking at him and his active lifestyle, I knew whatever he was doing was working.

The first night after getting my dreaded diagnosis, I needed to talk to someone who understood what I was going through, and more important, someone who was doing well. I gave Buzz a call.

"Tell me everything you are doing," I said, anxious to emulate him. "I'm taking notes."

The first thing he told me was to keep fighting and remain positive. He also told me about his strong spiritual connection, healthy diet, and exercise routine. I started following his advice as I went through ten months of chemotherapy.

I made significant changes in my lifestyle. I left my stressful job and made exercise, prayer, visualization, and affirmations a daily routine. I consulted regularly with my spiritual coach Terry McBride, an author and inspirational speaker I met at my church. I abandoned my chronic sugar addiction and switched to a healthy, whole foods diet. I focused on serving others in my breast cancer support group and at church. I also delivered meals to elderly people in my neighborhood. I began to devote more time to enriching all of my relationships, especially with my family, myself, and God.

Although my side effects were minimal and my tumors shrank with every scan, I fought off depression and was haunted by the sinking feeling I was going to die. With all the focus on myself and getting well, I felt useless and empty. I was searching for meaning in my life.

My husband Mike and I work in public relations and have always dreamed of writing a book together. He suggested I write a book about my cancer journey. "How can I write about it when I'm so early in the process?" I'd say.

In June, three months into my chemo treatments, we went on vacation with Mike's family at Rice Lake in Canada. On one of my daily morning walks, an idea popped into my mind. "Why not write a book about other advanced stage cancer patients and how they beat the odds?" I thought it would not only be therapeutic for me, but it could help others. I knew from experience that people needed to hear success stories and the importance of hope in fighting cancer. The empty hole I was feeling started to dissipate. This was the sense of purpose I was seeking.

I knew there had to be people out there like Buzz, and I was determined to find them. I began with a Web site that connects authors and reporters to sources. Later I contacted the Lance Armstrong Foundation, which publicized my call for stories in one of their newsletters. I started a blog to share stories and ask for more. I networked on Twitter and Facebook and carried business cards for my blog, talking up my project wherever I went.

The more people I found who shared their stories, the more confident I became that I, too, would beat the odds. I talked with so many of these incredible survivors that it began to seem they were the norm, not the exception to it. They showed me anything is possible, and there is always hope.

As I write this, I am continuing treatment for cancer with hormone therapy, diet, supplements, exercise and prayer. My latest scans show my efforts are working. The spots are shrinking and showing reduced cancer activity.

For me, cancer was a wake-up call. If I didn't learn the first time around, this second bout certainly caught my attention. Cancer has brought many blessings that I would not have realized without this daunting challenge. Writing this book is certainly one of them. The process of interviewing the amazing individuals featured in this book and writing their stories has been extremely therapeutic.

This book is for people who need proof that advanced cancer doesn't have to be a death sentence...even if that's what doctors predict. The outstanding individuals who share their stories in the following pages prove you cannot place a time limit on the human spirit. They simply refused to give up and accept a doctor's prediction on how long they had to live.

These miracle survivors taught me cancer doesn't have to be a death sentence. From them, I learned cancer was the beginning of a new way of life filled with appreciation, hope, and discovering my potential. I hope reading *From Incurable to Incredible* will inspire you to overcome your obstacles—whatever they might be.

Visit Tami at her blog, *Miracle Survivors: Inspiration and Information for Cancer Thrivers*, at www.miraclesurvivors.com.

CHAPTER 2

I'm here for a reason

Greg Barnhill

Age 56
Intraocular melanoma and mesothelioma
Diagnosed 2001 and 2004
Houston, Texas

I'm an insurance investigator. My job involves surveying damage from disasters—whether it's a natural one like a hurricane or man-made such as the Oklahoma City bombing. I wouldn't think twice about walking on a roof or stepping through rubble from a fire. I thought I'd seen it all. But that was before cancer.

I started seeing flashes in my left eye after being on the scene for Tropical Storm Allison. I figured it was stress-related, but I decided to go to my eye doctor just in case. He looked at it and said there was something wrong in the back of my eyeball. So I went to a retina specialist who ran some tests. He told me, "You have a lesion under the optic nerve. It's cancer."

My tumor was in an unusual place—the incident rate is six per million people or 1,400 cases a year. How I got it, no one knows. I suspect the culprit was creosote (the black, grimy stuff that's on telephone poles) that splashed in my eye when I was working on a high school Boy Scout project.

My doctor recommended a treatment where they implanted a small, gold plaque infused with radioactive seeds behind the eye. I was in the hospital almost a week over Christmas while I recovered from the surgery. Later I had another surgery to remove the radioactive plaque. Despite some loss of vision, I was fine. But I was told to do regular checkups because this kind of cancer often spreads to the liver.

In 2003, they said the tumors were growing again, but luckily it was contained in the eye. Removing my eye was my only option. Thanks to the wonders of medical technology, they were able to connect some donor tissue to the muscles behind the eye so my prostheses can move normally. People don't even notice.

I continued my checkups without incident until a year later. Soon after my regular scans, my doctor called and said he needed to see me to go over my results. When it's good news, they tell you over the phone. When it's bad news, they want to tell you in person. He wanted to meet in his faculty office before rounds.

My wife Sue went with me, and we were a wreck as we sat there waiting. The doctor told us, "We found lesions in your abdomen when we were doing the ultrasound. We're not sure what they are. We can watch them, or we can do a biopsy."

I said I didn't want to wait, so we did the biopsy. We found out it was mesothelioma, a rare cancer caused by asbestos exposure. Typically it's in your lungs; mine was in the omentum, a layer of muscle that covers the liver and abdomen.

Somewhere down the line, I'd been exposed. Before I was diagnosed, I never thought about the dangers of my job. When a building burned down, I never thought of what might be floating around in the air while I was walking around. I began taking precautions from that moment on.

My doctor recommended a clinical trial at the National Cancer Center and National Institutes of Health in Maryland for a new treatment called CHPP, which stands for Continuous Hyperthermic Peritoneal

Perfusion. The surgical procedure involves heating the chemotherapy drugs and distributing them throughout the peritoneal cavity wall.

They told me, "This is not a curable cancer, but maybe we can manage it." At that time, depending on what you read, the mortality rate was eight-and-a-half to eighteen months. I was told it was caught relatively early. If I hadn't been getting regular follow-ups, they would have found it much later.

The surgery alone lasted eleven hours. Surgeons removed my omentum, spleen, and tumors, then inserted a port into my abdomen for the chemo drugs. It took another hour and a half to wrap me in ice while they circulated the heated drugs throughout my peritoneal cavity.

Ten days after the surgery, they did another round of chemo through my port—this time while I was awake. When I came home after a couple of weeks in the hospital, my incision was still open so an infection I'd developed could heal. This took almost six months. Sue was amazing. She became my caregiver, packing my incision and changing dressings twice a day. We also received a lot of support from people at church and work.

In 2008, the doctor at the National Cancer Institute released me from the clinical trial. He said, "You're ahead of the curve; what we did is now the standard of care for this disease. You don't have to come back anymore." I've been in remission ever since.

Although the odds were against me, I think statistics are what you make of them. It's like politicians from opposing parties – they can both say the same things, but in different ways. A really good article about how statistics can be skewed is called, "The Median Isn't the Message" by Dr. Stephen Jay Gould, a mesothelioma survivor. It helped confirm my belief that cancer doesn't have to be a death sentence. New research and treatments are coming out all the time. My clinical trial couldn't have been done twenty years ago.

I've had two rare diseases. Now to be alive and well – it's a miracle. From the fall of 2001 to December 2006, I've had seven surgeries. I have no gallbladder, spleen, omentum, or left eye, but thanks to the man upstairs taking good care of me, I'm here. I believe it's for a reason.

My faith had a lot to do with my survival. There have been times when I was lying in the hospital bed feeling angry and asked, "God what do I do?" I eventually realized there is a purpose for everything.

That purpose, for me, is to help others who have cancer. I volunteer for a group called Lifeline Chaplaincy and see cancer patients and their caregivers at local hospitals. We talk to patients and families and see how we can help meet their needs, whether it's finding accessible parking or serving them communion. I go to the chemo ward on my lunch hour every Friday to see who's there and talk to them. They'll ask questions about getting a second opinion and talking to their kids about cancer. I don't give advice; I just let them talk.

I also volunteer for an organization called CanCare, which partners cancer survivors with others who have the same diagnosis and life circumstances. Recently a CanCare coordinator told me about a lady in the hospital who'd been diagnosed with peritoneal mesothelioma: "She doesn't know if she wants to talk to anyone yet. She's pretty upset. Would you talk to her?" So I went there and we talked. Usually people are shocked and overwhelmed when they're first diagnosed.

It helps to meet someone who can say, "Been there, done that, got the T-shirt, and now I'm fine."

Had you told me five or six years ago I'd be doing hospital ministry, I'd have said you were crazy. It was the farthest thing from my mind. But I've read we all have gifts and we should use them. Mine is compassion, and until now, I didn't realize I had it. If this building burned down, I could tell you what you'd need to rebuild it. That's not a gift, it's a skill. Compassion is a gift. I know what it's like to lie there wondering if you're going to live or die. Some of the patients I see don't get any visitors because they're from out of town. I can be there and let them know someone cares and understands.

At our church, when someone is diagnosed with cancer, people say, "Go talk to Greg." I keep a case of Lance Armstrong Foundation notebooks and other materials for that purpose. I meet with them and give them a book. I tell them, "It's going to be okay. Cancer's not the end of the world; it's beatable. Look at me." I'm blessed to be able to tell people that.

Lifeline Chaplaincy: www.lifelinechaplaincy.org
CanCare: www.cancare.org

CHAPTER 3

Erasing the stigma of lung cancer

Deb Violet

Age 55
Stage IIIA lung cancer
Diagnosed 1998
Augusta, Maine

I'm very independent. I've lived in Maine my whole life, and I think Maine people are like that; sometimes to a fault. It was very hard at first to let people in when I was sick. I just wanted to hide it.

I was forty-four when I was diagnosed. I was given a 10 percent chance of living two years. It was quite a while into my staging before I told my son and parents I was sick and might not make it. My stepfather was currently battling late stage prostate cancer and my mom was more than ten years out from stage III colon cancer. I tried to carry the burden myself because I saw what my parents' diseases had done to them and my son, and I just didn't want to do that to them.

It was very difficult to go into work and tell my supervisors I was sick. I thought I'd be ostracized. When I was first diagnosed, people did stop coming by my desk to chat on Mondays. I finally went to them and said something. One person admitted, "I don't know what to say anymore." I told him to just ask about my weekend like he used to. It kind of broke the ice.

After that, I'd come into work and there'd be a card, a piece of fruit, or a flower on my desk. Every day, I'd look forward to the surprise sitting on my desk. Some people who reached out to me didn't even know me. I was working late and the night janitor came up and said, "My wife had breast cancer thirty years ago, and she's fine. You are going to be just fine as well."

I never asked for help. But when people asked if they could do something for me, I'd let them. People would come over and cook a meal and visit or invite me to functions. I never refused; I was very grateful people wanted me around them.

I realized this cancer wasn't just about me. It was about everyone who came into contact with me. And for them and me to get through it, I had to open up and let people in. I couldn't just think of myself; I had to focus on how it was affecting other people.

The support lifted me up throughout my long fight, which included chemotherapy, followed by surgery and radiation. God did the rest.

At one point, I felt like I was being put in a vise and it was being turned tighter and tighter. Everything that was on the Internet about lung cancer was very depressing. I remember one night I was out in the garden thinking about my terrible prognosis. This little voice in my head said, "Why are you focusing on the 90 percent of people who didn't make it; why don't you focus on the 10 percent who do?"

Looking back, God was trying to reach out to me, saying, "Don't worry about this; I'll see you through it." From that point on, I just knew everything was going to be okay.

With that peace of mind, I was ready to use my experiences to help others. Just as I was just recovering from my radiation, I started my advocacy work. While I was sick, I was constantly on the Internet looking for information, but learned there was hardly anything out there. One night I was watching a TV program that featured the Alliance for Lung Cancer Advocacy, Support and Education (later renamed the Lung Cancer Alliance.)

The very next day I called them and said I'd like to do something for Maine citizens. They sent me a start-up packet with clear ribbon pins to raise lung cancer awareness. I set up a booth at the local hospital and began passing out pins to doctors and patients. Someone from the thoracic oncology and surgery group stopped by and said they didn't know lung cancer had a recognized pin. Soon people from the pulmonary unit came and grabbed up the pins. They were so excited about it.

I soon realized that lung cancer has a very big stigma attached to it. There is so much support around breast, colon, and prostate cancer, but not for lung cancer. Lung cancer is underfunded, too. For every lung cancer death, only $1,300 goes toward lung cancer research. For breast cancer it's $20,000 to $23,000; prostate, $18,000. So our outcomes are not as great as other kinds of cancers. Other cancers are underfunded, like pancreatic cancer, but without the stigma.

Even though I quit smoking three years before I was diagnosed, I felt blamed for my disease. At times I blamed myself. When I'm doing public speaking, the first thing people ask is how long did I smoke. If people aren't smokers, they seem to breathe a sigh of relief that they won't get lung cancer.

I work hard to get more support and recognition of lung cancer. Sometimes it makes me very unpopular. For years, I worked to persuade the governor of Maine to proclaim November Lung Cancer Awareness Month. About a year ago, I asked one of the senators to sponsor a bill to make this a law. Ed Miller from the American Lung Cancer Association and I testified before the committee. They came back and said they just wanted one week as Cancer Awareness Week; they wouldn't acknowledge lung cancer. We eventually convinced them to proclaim November 1 as Lung Cancer Awareness Day, but not without a fight.

Someone from the committee asked me what I wanted. I replied, "It isn't what I want, but what I want for the *citizens of Maine*. I want them to be recognized and to have support, compassion, better treatment options and survival rates for lung cancer."

Maine is a very poor state, with a very high unemployment and school dropout rate. There's a lot of smoking and alcoholism. Maine residents need to have good healthcare.

The state has done very well in lung cancer prevention and smoking cessation programs. With all the smoking programs we have in place, teenage smoking has dropped 50 percent. I testified last year to create a bill making it illegal to smoke in cars transporting children under the age of eighteen. I think Maine is the second state in the nation to pass a law like that.

We are making strides trying to prevent lung cancer, but 16 percent of all new lung cancer cases are nonsmokers. These nonsmokers account for more than 16,000 lung cancer deaths per year in the U.S. That's more than ovarian cancer or lymphoma.

I've traveled all over the country to attend meetings of various cancer and medical organizations. I love to travel; I've been to Israel, Egypt, Hong Kong, and China for vacations. I would love to be a nomad and travel everywhere and experience things I learned about in school. My advocacy work gives me more opportunities to travel in the U.S. Whenever I go to a conference, I always arrive a couple of days early to explore the city. If I hadn't had cancer, I probably wouldn't have done that until I retired.

I feel there was a reason I had lung cancer. I could have had any other kind of cancer; my family has a history of cancer. Why did I get it, and why did I survive? I think it was so I could give back to society, help people with this disease, speak up and give them encouragement that they, too, can survive.

Nobody talks about lung cancer, so nobody knows people survive lung cancer. People gave to me in my time of need and were so open and caring. I want to give back to the people of Maine.

I still have lung problems; my doctor says I have chronic pulmonary lung disease. I've had some scares like when I came back from China with pneumonia, but I'm really too busy to worry.

I wake up in the morning and thank God for the day because every day is a blessing. And when I crawl in bed at night, I thank God for the day, no matter how good or bad it was. Cancer has blessed me to be able to do that.

This sounds kind of odd, but I would not want to die without experiencing the love, caring, and nurturing I received during my cancer treatments. If I have inspired others and given them hope, I know my work is well worth it.

Lung Cancer Alliance: www.lungcanceralliance.org

CHAPTER 4

Living for two

Cathy Winebrenner Wolfe

Age 38
Ovarian cancer
Diagnosed mid 1997 and late 1997
Indianapolis, Indiana

I come from a large family. When I was nine, my dad and stepmother opened Winebrenner's Restaurant. My four brothers and I grew up together working there; it was a lot of fun. We definitely had our share of arguments and disagreements as children. But as grown-ups, my brothers and I are closer than anybody could have dreamed.

I wanted what I had as a child for my own family. When Pat proposed to me, I told him, "Don't put that ring on my finger unless you want ten children!"

Pat and I married in 1994 and had Christopher, our "honeymoon baby," about nine months later. It was very important for me to stay home with my child, so I started a licensed daycare business. When I became pregnant again two years later, we were excited to have our children two years apart. They could be friends; it would be wonderful!

Everything was going fine until late into the first trimester when I miscarried. It was a profoundly difficult experience for me.

Several months after the baby would have been born, I was pregnant again. We had our first clue when I started buying my crave food—bags of frozen egg rolls with sweet and sour sauce.

After doing my blood work, the doctor discovered I didn't have enough progesterone to maintain the pregnancy. So I started artificial progesterone treatments to avoid losing another child. Soon after, I was at the park with my daycare children when I started having severe cramps. I was terrified it was another miscarriage. A friend who lived nearby came out to help when she saw me writhing in pain on a picnic table.

At the emergency room, they performed an ultrasound. The baby was just a speck at that point. Based on all my blood work, I still had a pregnancy. Then the technician blurted out, "My God! I've never seen a cyst this large on a woman, let alone a pregnant woman!"

I was terrified. The doctor immediately stormed out of the room, obviously unhappy with the tech. He came back in and told me they were unable to determine exactly what it was at that time. However, I did have a nine-centimeter cyst on my ovary.

By the time I returned the following week, the cyst had grown to fourteen centimeters, squeezing the fetus from the left. My doctor thought it was a corpus luteum cyst, a harmless cyst which releases hormones to prepare the body for pregnancy. He estimated it would dissipate by the ninth week of pregnancy. But soon, they found another tumor on the ovary: both tumors were growing rapidly. By the sixth week of my pregnancy, I had collapsed from pain because the tumors were pressing on my organs. As we approached the nine-week mark, I was admitted into the hospital for pain. They told me these could be dermoid tumors, saclike growths comprised of hair, fluid, teeth, or skin glands that sometimes appear in pregnancy.

I decided to seek another opinion and found Dr. Olive Soriero, a renowned gynecological oncologist. I called her office, and got an appointment 7:30 the next morning.

Pat was caring for Christopher and my daycare children, so I went alone. Dr. Soriero said she had only seen two other cases like mine in all of her years of practice. I replied, "I want to have ten children, and I'm here so you can help me continue this pregnancy."

She looked over the top of her glasses at me, then she told me point-blank she thought it was ovarian cancer, which is very rare during pregnancy. My only guarantee for survival would be to have a hysterectomy that day or the next day. I immediately fell apart.

After I pulled myself together, I had to drive to the hospital to have more tests. I don't remember the drive at all. They put me in the triage room and I was so hysterical, screaming and crying, that they moved me to a private room. I called my grandma, mom, and best friend Wendy, but I didn't know how to tell Pat. Wendy left work to come to the hospital to be with me.

Wendy calmed me down enough so she felt I could safely drive myself home. When I walked in, Pat could tell I had a very rough day. He just held me, asking, "What's wrong, Cathy?" Finally I told him what happened.

He called his mother, who's a nurse and lives out of town. She and Pat's sisters arrived about two hours later. She had contacted my doctor and arranged for us to have a consultation the following morning.

Dr. Soriero is extremely honest. I admire her for not sugarcoating the truth, but it was a very gloomy conversation. She told me, "I can guarantee your survival if you have surgery today or tomorrow. After that, there are no guarantees."

I pleaded, "But is there any way to go day by day and give this baby a little bit more strength to guarantee his or her survival?" I knew a baby needed twenty-seven weeks to survive being born prematurely. She told me, "You'll never make it to twenty-seven weeks."

I begged her to do whatever it took to get me there. She finally relented. "You are putting me in a very difficult position," she said. "If you went to ten different doctors and told them what you wanted to do, they would all most likely refuse to treat you."

She agreed to continue with the pregnancy because she knew I was willing to do whatever it took. We had ultrasounds twice a week. I saw my child smile, turn over and suck his thumb. This gave me more motivation than ever to continue my pregnancy.

The pain was unbearable, so she prescribed morphine and Vicodin, which I took around the clock. At that point, it was the only way I could continue the pregnancy. She wanted me to consult with a neonatologist about delivering a premature baby addicted to painkillers, just in case. That was heartwrenching, but I told myself I'd rather have a baby addicted to painkillers than no baby at all.

I was unable to keep food down and survived on ice chips and water. The tumors were getting so big that any fall or pressure could cause them to rupture. Dr. Soriero likened it to a dandelion. When you blow on the seeds, they go wherever they want. So I was confined to a wheelchair.

When the tumors began obstructing my bowel, my husband gave me treatments every day. Pat was very involved with helping taking care of Christopher, too. He did whatever needed to be done. He is a wonderful man!

Thank goodness we had help. My neighbor came every day to take care of Christopher while Pat was working. She wouldn't accept a penny for it. My stepmother came down from Michigan every other weekend.

There were family and friends who disagreed with our decision. We received cards from friends and strangers and roses from a family member with messages that said, "Cathy, we love you. Please have the surgery."

I could understand their concern. I was scared; I knew my life was at risk. But I decided I wasn't going to wake up every day of my life angry because someone talked me into something I didn't want to do. My husband and I needed to make this decision on our own.

I prayed for courage and strength. I prayed for the baby to survive. I wanted to be a mother so much. It felt like my purpose in life. I fought hard because I wanted to give this baby a chance. I knew I would be a great mom, and that gave me strength.

At about thirteen weeks, Dr. Soriero told me, "Cathy, I have a feeling I'll be holding your baby soon." I knew that meant surgery was inevitably close.

At fifteen weeks, I felt like I was dying. I was rushed to the hospital where they found my potassium levels were dangerously low. My body was starting to become toxic from a bowel obstruction. The cysts had gotten so big they were crowding out the baby. They hooked me up to a lot of IVs and pumped me with antibiotics and nutrients. I prayed, holding my rosary the whole time.

When my blood levels stabilized, they called Dr. Soriero to lead the surgery. During the procedure, she gently held my uterus with one hand while removing the tumors. That alone could have caused me to go immediately into labor. The smallest one was twenty-two centimeters, much larger than the fetus at that time.

About five and half hours later, I woke up back in my room. The first thing I said was, "Baby?" Pat said, "Yes." Then I said, "Cancer?" He said I'd have to ask the doctor. I knew my baby had survived and was so very happy.

I later learned that although they removed the cancer, it would probably recur because what remained of my ovaries would be seeded. I was in the hospital about two weeks, then went home to recover and wean off my medication.

Miraculously, I carried my son to term, delivering him on November 6, 1997. He was healthy and perfect, and we named him Johnathan. Soon after he was born, Pat leaned over him and said, "Welcome to our world. It's okay, Mommy and Daddy are here." At that moment, Johnathan reached his hands up to Pat's face. What a beautiful moment!

I was enjoying motherhood, hoping to have another child, until December 1997. That's when I went back for a checkup and learned my cancer returned. Once again, I was told I needed a hysterectomy.

I was extremely distraught. I drove around for four hours on country roads looking for a deer, seeing that as a sign to have the surgery. I asked God, "Please just let me see a deer. That'll be the sign that everything will be okay. It would give me peace with this decision." There was no deer. But later that night, as Pat and I were leaving for dinner, a deer ran by my car. I was so happy; this was the sign that I was making the right decision.

I had the hysterectomy in February of 1999. I have been clear of cancer since then. Dr. Soriero said that five years ago, Johnathan wouldn't have survived, and ten years ago neither one of us would have. I am blessed to have a doctor who supported me and continues to support me to this day.

Today, I am helping other women in my situation by volunteering for Hope for Two, an organization that provides information, support, and hope to women diagnosed with cancer while pregnant. They match people up with the same cancers. Although there aren't a lot of pregnant ovarian cancer patients, I've talked to several through the group. The last woman I spoke with lives in the Philippines.

Christopher's fifteen now and only remembers some of what happened. He used to worry; but today he knows Mom is going to be fine. Johnathan is almost thirteen, and we who love him can't imagine life without him. He's happy to be alive and comfortable in his own skin. He recently wrote a paper for school on what freedom means to him. He related how his most important freedom is the gift of life. He described how his Mommy gave him that when she was pregnant with cancer and fought to save us both.

I understand what Johnathan is saying; I certainly feel freer than ever before. This experience has changed forever who I am as a person. It makes the little things seem nonexistent. I know what the big obstacles can be; I've already climbed that mountain. I am thankful for each and every day.

Hope for Two: www.hopefortwo.org

CHAPTER 5

Give Strong

Penny Feddick

Age 40
Stage IV non-Hodgkin lymphoma
Diagnosed 2002
Tucson, Arizona

It was the chance of a lifetime. In 2002, the Lance Armstrong Foundation (LAF) chose me to travel to Washington, D.C. with Lance and representatives from every state to fight for cancer funding and survivors' rights. I represented Arizona and met with Senator John McCain. Two of the top LAF staff came with me since this was the time leading up to his presidential campaign.

Sen. McCain did not seem responsive to our position, so I said to him, "You don't know how much I spread this word. I have a big voice in my community, and I'm not going to shut up when I go back home."

He responded that he was not on the appropriations committee, so there wasn't a lot he could do. I looked at him and said, "One in two men die from cancer; one in three women will die from it. You've already had it, so which one of you will die?"

He replied, "Boy, you're a feisty little one!" I later received a nice letter from him, but it was kind of frustrating and a real eye-opener for me.

When I was diagnosed with stage IV non-Hodgkin lymphoma at age thirty-four, I never thought I would be standing before a presidential candidate fighting for cancer reform. My focus then was fighting for my life.

My oncologist, Dr. Taetle, recommended I see a bone marrow specialist. So I went with my stepfather to University Medical Center. She told me I needed to be put on an international transplant list, and I was going to die within a year if I didn't get one. I was adopted, so I didn't know my family heritage. I knew this hurt my chances of finding a donor.

I freaked out. I went over to the oncology center and said, "I want to see Dr. Taetle now!" When he took us back to his office, I asked why he didn't tell me I only had a year to live. He said, "Because I don't think you are going to die within a year. We can treat this with Rituxan. Can you start chemo tomorrow?" And that's what I did.

The doctor told me I would lose my hair with chemo. I was a little upset. I always had this big Texas hair, and I was really proud of it. So my girlfriends picked me up in a convertible and we had what we called, "Wigging Out Day." I think all girlfriends or family members should do this for a person. We tried on wigs, wore big feather boas and sunglasses, and went out for margaritas and chips. They said, "We can talk about cancer or not talk about cancer. Today is your day."

I was doing chemo eight hours a day, five days a week, with only a week off every three weeks. So as soon as I started to feel good, I had to go back in again. This was very hard because I was always a very active person: I was a swimmer and a runner and I always took trips with my girlfriends. I was used to being the life of the party, but with chemo, all I wanted to do was sleep. This went on for three years, and we never could find a match for a bone marrow transplant.

One night when it was all becoming too much for me, I went to church and prayed. I gave it all to God and said, "I can't handle this by myself anymore. I need help." I envisioned that God had His hand around the cancer, and it wasn't going to spread.

The next day, I went to the doctor to get my scan results. He gave me a hug. I fearfully asked if something was wrong. He said, "No. Your scan is showing no cancer. What did you do?" I was blown away by this extraordinary news, but I knew the answer. I responded, "I went to God and gave it all to Him."

That was four years ago, and I've been free of cancer ever since. I cried when I completed chemo because I had spent so much time with my oncologist, nurses, and fellow patients. My doctor treated me as a person and a friend. He did not treat me like a number, like I was going to die. He's just hilarious. He calls me "trouble with a capital T."

I always carry the petition for the National Call to Action on Cancer with me in my car. I'm sending it to Lance, so when he goes to D.C. he can show that people are still concerned about it.

During my treatment, my mom bought me Lance Armstrong's book, *It's Not About the Bike*. I told my employer I wanted to participate in the LAF Ride for the Roses (now called the LIVESTRONG Challenge). The company paid for me to go. There were ten thousand people on the ride; it looked like a sea of yellow. I never saw so many people who were affected by cancer. That was the first time I broke down in tears because I realized how large this epidemic was.

From that point on, I became involved volunteering for LAF, as well as the Leukemia/Lymphoma Society, American Red Cross, and National Bone Marrow Registry. I worked hard to decrease the myth that bone marrow transplants are extremely painful. I asked people, "How many times do you have the chance to save someone's life?" As a result, about five hundred people donated.

With non-Hodgkin lymphoma, the seventh year, which is this year, is usually when it comes back. You're always looking over your shoulder. I still get scanned regularly. When I'm lying there getting a scan, I get anxious because you never know if a cough or migraine is due to the disease. There's nothing I can do about it; that worry is probably going to be there for the rest of my life.

One worry is that they have never found a bone marrow match for me. But I keep telling myself it's not going to come to that. Maybe I'm being naive, but I believe you can keep cancer at bay by having a positive attitude, setting goals, and acting like it's not going to kill you. I wear a pin that says "PIE." It stands for passion, intensity, and enthusiasm, and that's how I live my life.

It's been hard on my parents because they think I'm going to eventually die from this. I don't believe that. I believe God gave me this disease as a purpose. Volunteering for the cause is my passion. I've always been very direct and vocal; I can do for other cancer patients what they can't do for themselves. I pick them up if they need a ride and bring them meals. There are about five people who have called me and said, "I don't know who else to talk to, but I can call you."

This year will be the second annual LIVESTRONG Day, a run, walk, and ride I've organized in Tucson. It's a day of celebration; a chance to raise awareness and funds for cancer. I recently met with the mayor to organize the LIVESTRONG at School program. It goes from kindergarten up to college and provides ways to answer students' questions, such as, "Why is my teacher wearing a wig this year?" or "Why do my parents fight about cancer?"

When I volunteer, I get back a hundredfold. I come away with the most amazing experiences. I've made some of the best friends in the world, and it helps me to stay focused and busy. I continue to get people to sign petitions, and I write monthly letters to my senators. I've even written to President Obama. I stay on them. They know who I am.

American Red Cross: www.redcross.org
Lance Armstrong Foundation: www.livestrong.org
Leukemia/Lymphoma Society: www.lls.org
National Call to Action on Cancer Prevention and Survivorship: www.nctacancer.org
National Bone Marrow Registry: www.marrow.org

Purpose

Discussion Questions

1. What gave the individuals featured in Part I a sense of purpose?
2. Do you feel having a sense of purpose has an impact on survival? Why or why not?
3. What gives you a sense of purpose in your life?
4. Has having cancer or having a loved one with cancer changed your views about how you live your life with purpose?
5. Organizations often have mission statements to describe their purpose for doing business. If you were to develop a personal mission statement, what would it be?

Part II
Attitude

CHAPTER 6

Winning the big game

Bob Kiesendahl

Age 39
Chronic mylogeneous leukemia (CML)
Diagnosed 1998
Hawley, Pennsylvania

For fifty years our family has owned and managed a destination family resort located in the Pocono Mountains in northeastern Pennsylvania. It's where I grew up and where I now work. My childhood was great. My brothers and I were outdoors all the time—active on the lake and playing sports. It was the best of both worlds—we were in a beautiful, rural setting with all the facilities and activities of the resort, plus friends and family members around us.

At age twenty-eight, I was still living this idyllic lifestyle. I was healthy, athletic, and working full-time in my family's business. My wife Jen and I had recently married. I felt invincible.

I can still remember the fateful call when my family doctor explained that the excruciating pain I was experiencing in my hip was from my white blood cell counts, which were through the roof. That was an indicator of leukemia. My world came crashing in.

I didn't even know what leukemia was, but I would learn very quickly. I had chronic mylogeneous leukemia (CML), a type of leukemia that statistically occurs more often in very young children or older adults. My disease was in a blastic phase, which meant it was spreading very quickly. I was given a 25 percent chance to survive—and that was *with* a bone marrow transplant. At that time, it was the only chance I had.

Right up front, Jen and I had a serious talk. I told her, "I don't know what the outcome is going to be. You're a young person and have your whole life to live. I respect whatever decision you make." She told me, "No, I'm staying." I respect and love her even more for her strength and commitment to stand by me as I fought cancer.

My family members were tested as possible donors, with no luck. My brothers, who were the most likely donors, matched each other perfectly, but not me. We then turned to the National Bone Marrow Registry, which matches donors with patients. Within a few months, the registry was able to find a good match who was willing to donate.

My oncologist at the Penn State Hershey Medical Center recommended I go to the Fred Hutchinson Cancer Research Center in Seattle, a facility that pioneered bone marrow transplantation. My wife and mom went with me as caregivers. Before we left, I sat with them and the rest of my family and told them, "I don't want to see any tears, negativity, or anything in the way of pity. I want everyone to be upbeat and positive. We're going to get through this." They abided by my wishes and were incredibly strong for me.

I spent a little over four months in Seattle. I had full-body radiation and aggressive chemo to knock everything out of my system. On May 14, 1999, I had my transplant. I now consider this date my second birthday.

Compared to the physical regiment I went through previously, the transplant itself was anticlimactic; it simply dripped in through my port. The high anxiety kicked in again afterwards as we waited to see if my counts would come back after totally knocking out my immune system.

The days moved slowly. I tried to stay as determined and stuck to a routine each day. I would wake up, eat, at a certain time. I requested an exercise bike and pumped away while listening to Pearl Jam or watching TV. This was good for me mentally and physically.

Having an athletic background, I placed my battle into a simple sports model. All my pre-transplant treatments—the radiation and chemo—were my practices and training for the big game. The transplant was my personal Super Bowl. I was going to play as hard as I could and win.

I did some visualization of what was happening to my body. I viewed all the unpleasant side effects from the treatments as proof that the cancer cells were leaving my body and dying. I also focused on where I wanted to be when I regained my life. It wasn't a matter of *if* I was going to survive, it was *when* I survived. And I knew when this was all over; I wanted to do something to help others affected by cancer.

At the time, there were no beds on the adult transplant floor, so I was placed on the pediatric floor. Most of the children were cancer patients; many were transplant patients. I was humbled by them—always smiling and resilient. The kids inspired me with their innocence and strength.

One of the rules on the pediatric floor was that when you were able, you had to start exercising by walking the halls. They made us do as many laps as our age. I would always joke with the kids that they had it easy—I was twenty-nine at the time.

There was another reason to fight this with everything I had. Having a family was one of the things I looked forward to most in life. Doctors told Jen and me that sterility was imminent after full-body radiation and intense chemotherapy. We followed suggestions to bank my sperm for the future. So imagine our surprise when we found we were expecting our first child just before I had my transplant!

Eventually my counts started to climb—my transplant took. I had some bumps along the way, but fortunately I progressed and was out of the hospital after thirty-four days.

I thought a successful transplant was "winning the Super Bowl," but I have been blessed with many more victories in my life. My wife and I today have three healthy boys. After our first son Zachary, we attempted invitro fertilization four times. During one of the attempts, we tragically lost twins who were born prematurely. We remained committed and fortunately received the blessing of our second son Luke as the result of our fourth attempt.

My third son Drew was a total surprise. Two years ago, Jen told me she was pregnant, but this time it happened by natural means. I was no longer sterile!

I couldn't believe it nor could my oncologist. "You continue to amaze me," he said as he shook his head. It showed us how life can turn around quickly. I had three miracle boys in my life, each with a unique story.

Another victory was being able to meet my donor. The National Bone Marrow Registry doesn't allow you to have contact with your donor immediately. After a year, you are allowed to send an anonymous letter with information about yourself. The letter cannot contain much detail, and the recipient has the option of whether or not to respond.

My donor Drew didn't respond for the first couple of months. Finally, we received a call. Drew, who was in the Air Force at the time, decided to participate in its bone marrow drive because he felt it would be a "good thing to do." He stepped in—a total stranger—and saved my life.

We have developed an amazing bond. Jen and I even named our third son after him. Our families have vacationed together in South Carolina, and he and his family come up every fall to our resort. I told him they have an open invitation to vacation here any time they want. It's the least I can do; how do you repay someone who saved your life?

From the beginning, I felt an obligation to help find a cure and give back to others. This helped provide me with inspiration to get through the treatments, transplant, and recovery. It was empowering to start thinking that way beyond my immediate situation.

I've been fortunate that our family business provides me with resources to raise money for the cause. Over the past nine years, my mother (a breast cancer survivor) and I have organized several grassroots fundraising efforts on our property. These include an annual golf tournament, 5K run, and other events, which have raised more than $400,000 for cancer centers and foundations. The support of my family, friends, and local businesses has been overwhelming.

I try to be that beacon of hope for others stricken with cancer. Not a week goes by that I don't get one or two phone calls asking me to talk to someone who has just been diagnosed. I tell them I survived pretty grim odds, and that they can too. By sharing my story, I can say, "Cancer rearranges your priorities in life and puts things in perspective."

I tell them how my cancer has never left me. It may have left my body, but it is always in the back my head. I have chosen to embrace how the experience has changed me for the better, not what it has taken from me.

I've resumed my normal lifestyle, remaining active and working. I don't take medication and just have routine six-month checkups with my oncologist. I cherish my boys and wife and all that I have. I realize I'm fortunate. Life can change quickly without warning. As a cancer survivor, I will continue to do all that I can to help others beat this disease.

National Bone Marrow Registry: www.marrow.org

CHAPTER 7

Finding the gift in cancer

Brenda Michaels

Age 60
Cervical and breast cancer
Diagnosed 1974, 1987 and 1988
Seattle, Washington

My first marriage was very abusive on both a physical and emotional level. It was not unlike how I was raised; our home life was a war zone most of the time. This was familiar to me. I married a man very much like my father.

I wasn't concerned about my spiritual life. If something happens to you, you blame somebody else. I wasn't in the position to take responsibility for my life. That's what I believed. I never questioned anything to see what I had to learn from the experience.

When I was twenty-six years old, I was diagnosed with cervical cancer. I had a hysterectomy, and they told me if it didn't come back five years later, I was cancer-free.

I stayed with my first husband for a few more years, then we divorced. I was single for awhile and still leading a high-drama, very unhealthy lifestyle. When I met my current husband, Rob, I was having dreams about being in Hollywood. The one dream I had repeatedly was that I was a talk show host. This fueled my desire to get into acting.

We moved to Hollywood. Rob became a producer, and I began acting in soap operas and commercials. All I cared about was how I looked. I was always thin and athletic and had good energy, so I ate what I wanted. I was drinking, smoking, consuming diet drinks, and eating a lot of red meat and sweets. None of it was organic.

Eight months after we moved and thirteen years after my cervical cancer diagnosis, I was diagnosed with cancer in my left breast. I noticed a lump, but was told it was just an infected milk duct. The doctor prescribed antibiotics, but that didn't help. It was two and a half years before I was diagnosed properly. Finally I went to a surgeon who did a needle biopsy, which confirmed it was cancer.

By then, it was too late to save my breast, so I had a mastectomy. I was fortunate it hadn't spread to the lymph system. They wanted to do chemo, but I refused. It did not feel right for me to go down that road.

I went to checkups and had blood drawn every three months. According to the oncologist, I was doing great, but I had concerns. I had a benign lump removed from my right breast years before the cervical cancer. There was scar tissue from that surgical procedure. I had read enough to know that scarring can leave calcium deposits that are actually malignant. I had a feeling this was the case for me, but I couldn't convince my surgeon.

A year after I lost my left breast, I had a routine mammogram on my right breast. Sure enough, it was cancer. I had another mastectomy, and tests revealed that this time it was in my lymph nodes.

My surgeon and my oncologist were adamant about doing chemotherapy. Again, I followed how I was really feeling in my body, and intuitively, it still did not feel right for me to do it. The prognosis, without chemotherapy, was very poor. My oncologist felt within a year

I would have major metastases. He said, "If that happens, there is nothing I can do for you." He was telling me I may have a year or so to live because, if this happened, I'd be in bad shape.

I had to make a big decision to either do chemo out of fear (which it would have been for me) or to find another way. I didn't have a clue what that was. I wanted to know why this cancer was active in my body. What was really going on? Neither of my doctors could tell me what was causing it. I wondered, "Is there something beyond my physical body? Is there something more to it than this?"

My oncologist released me when he learned I wouldn't do chemotherapy. He scolded me and said I was being foolish. He couldn't be responsible if this was what I wanted to do.

I went home and prayed. I surrendered to having symptoms of cancer in my body, that I had no idea what I was going to do, and that there was a good possibility I could die in a year or two. I owned up to a lot of things I was unwilling to claim and wrote it all down. It was the first time I had been that honest with myself in my life. By emptying out my soul in this way, it created a space for some solutions and answers.

There was a part of me that knew if I continued the way I had been, I was going to die and that chemotherapy was going to be a Band-aid for me and not an answer. I didn't ask God, "How do I cure this?" Of course I wanted to cure it, but I was more interested in healing my body and my life than curing it. I asked, "What do I do next?" Within two days, the doctor who ultimately led me to Dr. Nicolas Gonzalez, an immunology specialist who treats cancer in a holistic way, magically showed up in my life.

Dr. Gonzalez put me on a very restrictive diet that would give my body the nutrients and enzymes it needed to balance and thrive. I juiced three times a day and ate only organic food. I eliminated the toxic chemicals around me. I did sea salt and soda baths with purified water twice a week. I did it by the letter because I wanted to stay in integrity. It was a complete 180 degree turn for me.

The first seven months of the program I was sicker than a dog because my body was letting go of toxins. I had fevers, congestion, and exhaustion. My doctor told me these symptoms would happen, but just to be with it. As time went on, I started feeling better and better. I was thinking more clearly; it was like a fog had lifted. I was having deeper meditations and became more highly intuitive. All my senses were heightened.

But I went further than that. I began to look at the emotional and spiritual components of disease. It opened my eyes, and I had a profound awakening as a result.

I wanted to be the emotionally, mentally, and spiritually healthiest person I could be, and I wanted to share that with others. I never prayed, "God help me with this." I always prayed from the position that, "Okay God, this is what's happening. I'm asking for guidance, and I'm open to receive."

I received a strong message to start a gratitude book to focus on everything that was right in my life. I started feeling grateful for all the good in my life, including my cancer. In that moment, cancer was the right thing for me to be experiencing because it was part of my waking-up process.

I began to look at where I was stuffing my feelings rather than offending people in my life. I think every time you stuff your emotions, it is deposited somewhere in your body, imprinting into your cells. I believe this opens the door to illness, to cancer. Although there isn't any one cause, I think cancer happens when we're not dealing with our emotions or spiritual issues.

I began to develop my spiritual life, which led to becoming a minister, counseling cancer patients for nine years. One of the most common issues that came up with clients was control. It was certainly the case for me. I was always trying to control everything. It's incredibly fatiguing to try to control everything in life when in actuality there's no control. I realized that while I couldn't control events in my life, I *could* control my response to them. I could learn from it.

During this time, a friend of mine started a television show on public access in Los Angeles, which had a couple hundred thousand viewers. She asked me to join her. We produced and interviewed cutting-edge spiritual leaders. One of our very first interviews was Deepak Chopra, whose first book had just come out. About four years later, another friend of mine, who had a holistic, spiritually oriented radio show in LA, invited me to come on as a co-host.

This job gave me an idea for another show. Rob and I came up with a concept called, *Conscious Talk: Radio that Makes a Difference*. We decided to leave LA and start the show in Seattle, a city we felt would better match our holistic lifestyle.

Rob was in the television industry as a writer and producer for Aaron Spelling but had never been in front of the camera or on radio. Yet Rob and I were on the same spiritual path. Twenty years before I met him, Rob was diagnosed with non-Hodgkin lymphoma and was given a year to live. He went on a profound spiritual journey and found a doctor who put him on a regimen similar to mine. He's been cancer-free ever since. I invited him to co-host the show with me. It's worked out beautifully.

The show's purpose is to plant seeds of wisdom, hope, and inspiration, then give listeners the tools to make forward movement. The show is syndicated throughout the state of Washington and is on the Internet streaming live in the morning at www.conscioustalk.net. We're in 152 countries and also podcast our broadcasts. We've been on for eight years and have interviewed authors such as Marianne Williamson, Wayne Dyer, and Michael Beckwith on a variety of topics.

It took me a long time to come to peace with cancer. Fears still come up, and are very real. It's scary to look at what it's like to die. It takes a lot of courage, but we all have that reservoir of courage when we're willing to tap it. We do this by walking into what we fear the most and surrendering to it. People think if you surrender to cancer, it will kill you. But that's not true.

While meditating one day, I had a profound vision that I was presented with a gift box. When I took the ribbon off and opened it, the word, *cancer,* jumped out of the box. At that point, my mind got a hold of it and sparked all kinds of dark scenarios. When I finally went back into meditation and asked what it meant, I heard from that little voice deep inside that the cancer wasn't there to kill me. I was being given this gift to transform my life and, therefore, transmute this cancer.

That's when I was finally able to release the fear of dying. A miracle is merely a shift in perception. This was my miracle.

I still continue to juice and eat organic food, though I'm not as restrictive as I was initially. I still journal, do my gratitude book, pray, and meditate. I take responsibility for my life. I used to always have to be right as opposed to letting my spirit guide the ship. I'm not about being right anymore.

My health is the best it's ever been. Rarely do I get sick with anything. I truly believe that, given the proper environment on all levels, the body maintains a healthy status quo. It's like having a bank account. You have to have a certain amount saved to gain interest.

Twenty years since my third cancer, I remain cancer-free. I don't say, "I made it." I am constantly in a process of moving toward being a positive force on this planet.

Conscious Talk Radio: www.conscioustalk.net

CHAPTER 8

Prince for a day

As told by Paul and his mother Lisa

Paul Falk

Age 32
Acute myeloid leukemia
Diagnosed 1986 at age 9
Cincinnati, Ohio

isa: We had just returned from a trip to Disney World when we noticed his appetite was gone, and he was falling asleep at the dinner table. At first I attributed it to the strains of soccer practice and the start of school. Looking at his school picture taken at the time, we should have noticed something was wrong. He was so pasty, even though we just got back from Florida.

Paul: I woke up at about 2 A.M. to a whooshing sound. I couldn't figure out where it was coming from. Then I realized it was the sound of blood flowing through my ears. Being a curious kid, I lay in bed and held my breath. I felt my heart speed up and go faster and faster as the oxygen depleted in my lungs. I realized it was totally unnatural.

I went downstairs to tell Mom, and within a few hours, we were at the pediatrician's office.

Lisa: He was in a pool of sweat, but I tried to stay calm. The nurse noticed he had red dots up and down legs. The doctor was usually cool as a cucumber, but he anxiously said, "I don't know what's wrong. He might be bleeding internally." They sent us to another doctor down the street, padding our car with pillows and advising me to drive very slowly. "Don't let him cry," the doctor said. They were afraid he would have a stroke because his platelets were so low.

When we arrived, the pediatrician, two nurses, and a lab technician ran out the door. The doctor and nurse ushered us to the door. "I know it's cancer, but I don't know what type it is," the doctor told me. "In my thirty years as a pediatrician, I've never seen anything like this." We immediately went to Cincinnati Children's Hospital Medical Center.

The next day, a panel of fifteen doctors and healthcare professionals sat down with us and gave us the diagnosis: acute myeloid leukemia. It typically affects young adults from age seventeen to thirty, so it was unusual for a child to have it. It's an extremely violent cancer that forms in the blood marrow and moves very fast.

The doctors told us, "If Paul lives two weeks, we'll give him a month. If he lives a month, he might live three. If he lives three months, there's a good chance he'll survive six." They gave us the choice of standard treatment protocol or an experimental one called the Denver Protocol, which would be reviewed by doctors from around the country. We chose the latter.

Paul: I remember the first day I was in the hospital, I started shaking violently.

Lisa: When you give someone a lot of blood all at once, the body reacts to it. When he first started chemo, he was getting transfusions every day because his body wasn't producing blood. During his stay, he had sixty units of blood and forty-five units of platelets. They described his chemo treatment with a tree analogy. To kill the cancer, you have to prune the tree severely without killing it.

Paul: I was given a rather non-sugarcoated diagnosis on my first day at the hospital. Survival rates weren't discussed, but they explained what was wrong. I remember saying to the doctor, "It looks like I'm probably going to die."

Lisa: He told Paul, "Well if we have something to say about it, that's not going to be the case. But you have to fight, too."

Paul: I didn't really understand the meaning of death, but I knew it wasn't an option for me. I wasn't having any of it.

Lisa: We never talked about *not* getting better. We always talked about "*when* you get better." The staff at Children's Hospital believes in helping children understand what they need to do to get well. At every level, they let kids know what is going to happen to them. Paul wanted to participate. They used a teaching telescope to show him slides from his bone marrow harvest and taught him how to count his red blood cells.

Paul: It was supremely important to me to be able to walk around, but I couldn't since I was hooked up with IVs. We talked them into implanting a central line, which would allow me to move more freely. I developed an infection sometime during the procedure, but had no immunity to fight it. They told my parents I had twenty-four hours to live.

That night, I had a dream of sitting on a park bench with God and asking him why I was going through this. He said, "Because it's going to matter the rest of your life."

Lisa: He never shared this with us. But when he was going through that, I started praying the rosary. I dozed off and woke up at 2 A.M. There was a beautiful lady dressed in white and she was sponging Paul's head with a washcloth and murmuring to him softly.

I had this tremendous sense of peace, like *everything's going to be all right.* It was the first time I wasn't in a heightened state of stress. I just knew whatever happened; I'd have the strength to deal with it.

The next morning, Paul woke up and looked at the nurse. She asked if he was hungry, and he said, "Yeah, what's for breakfast?" She replied, "Whatever you want!" We knew then he was going to be all right.

We didn't discuss it for a year because I thought I was nuts. The woman in white obviously wasn't a nurse. I have a friend who prays to Mary. She came to see Paul in the hospital and said, "Wow! Can you smell that?" I apologized, saying it was probably the chemo and that Paul was getting sick a lot. "She said, "No, I smell roses. Mary has been here."

Paul: I was a very progress-oriented patient. I was concentrating on all the tangible results, controlling the things I was able to control. For example, they told me I had to eat. That's nonsense when they're putting all this toxic stuff into you. I remember throwing up a huge plate of lasagna they gave me. It looked like a massacre happened in my room.

Lisa: One of Paul's nurses, who was in the early stages of pregnancy, came to his room before his chemo and said, "We're premedicating you, so you need to have a nice meal beforehand. Would you like a bowl of chicken noodle soup?" He ordered spaghetti and meatballs, and she said, "Paul, please don't do that to me!" He folded his arms and said, "I know my rights, and if I want to have that and puke my guts up, you have to measure it! Too bad for you!"

Paul (laughing): They had me on drugs!

Lisa: He said, "I promise if you give me that, I won't throw up on your shift. I'll wait until the next one." I'd say to Paul, "That's awful of you; she's pregnant!"

Paul: I was just trying to eat what sounded good because it all tasted terrible. Everything tasted so off, it made me sick.

Lisa: After he completed chemo, Paul's body had to start producing blood to be released from the hospital. We said, "We've pruned the tree; let's start growing leaves!" Every day, we would pat his leg and say, "Come on bones, make some blood!" It must have worked because he was finally sent home after being in the hospital almost two months.

At home, Paul was able to see some of his friends from school, but with restrictions: they had to stay on the other side of the living room, and Paul wore a mask. One of his friends, Jeff, couldn't come over because he had cystic fibrosis and often developed lung infections that would kill Paul if he caught them.

Even before he became sick, Paul was always nice to kids who weren't well. Jeff couldn't run or play, so he'd be left out. Several times, Paul stayed in from recess to play with Jeff. That kindness paid off in a lot of ways. After Paul got better, Jeff received a dream from Cincinnati

Dreams Come True, which grants wishes to kids who are regular patients of Children's Hospital. Jeff told them, "Hey, I have a friend who needs a dream, too."

Paul: My dream was meeting President Reagan. They granted my wish, but we only spent a half a minute with him. We spent a lot of time, though, with George H.W. Bush who was then vice president. We met him in Canton, Ohio for the Football Hall of Fame induction and also met all the Most Valuable Players at the time. Then we flew to Washington, D.C. on Air Force Two with Vice President and Barbara Bush.

Lisa: He dunked cookies in milk on the plane with the vice president! Can you imagine that? They lost a child to leukemia, so they took a special interest in Paul. Bush made arrangements with the Secret Service to volunteer their own time to escort us all around Washington.

Two Secret Service agents drove us to see the U.S. Marine Corps Parade at the Iwo Jima monument. Just through the gate, a young Marine stopped our car. Our driver got out and talked to the Marine. We couldn't hear what they were saying, but the Marine told us to go on.

When we approached the long drive to the monument, every Marine stood at attention and gave us a salute. We asked why, and one of the agents told us, "When you're invited by the vice president of the United States, they pay attention. You're special."

Later, we had a private tour of the Air and Space Museum, and Paul was invited to target shoot at the FBI headquarters.

Paul: I shot a .357 Magnum pistol with the help of a trained professional. That thing could have thrown me back into the wall.

Lisa: He had a bruise on his chest.

Paul: And I didn't even care! That was one of the many amazing things we did. Months later on my birthday, we received a delivery from the White House.

Lisa: The FedEx driver was standing there with a package, his arms shaking and said, "I know this sounds presumptuous, but can I come in?" I asked why and he said, "I want to see what it is. It says it's from the vice president of the United States."

Paul: It was a personal letter from Vice President Bush with pictures of us with him, President Reagan, the director of the FBI, and in the cockpit of Air Force Two. Bush had a White House photographer follow us, shooting candid photos without our even knowing it.

Lisa: To thank him for his kindness, we mailed Vice President Bush some Cincinnati chili and a local brand of ice cream he liked. We sent enough for thirty-five people, but it first had to pass muster with the Secret Service. One day, one of the agents called and said, "Guess what we're doing, Paul? We're having chili!"

Paul: In retrospect, I'm glad I chose to go to Washington. A lot of kids who participated in the program asked for big-screen TVs and basketball courts for their yards. That would have been fun, but I had a remarkable experience.

I learned just how miraculous it was that I was able to go on the trip when I later went for my routine monthly checkup. It was a year since I was diagnosed, and we asked the doctor what happened to the other kids in the Denver Protocol. She told us ninety-seven had died, two were close to death, and one made it—that was me.

I believe I survived because I fought the disease and stayed positive. I understand now that even in grief and sorrow, God works through all of our experiences.

As a teenager, I fell into alcohol and drug addiction. From the time I was eighteen, I couldn't imagine living my life clean. In 2008, I got into trouble and spent some time in jail. I remember sitting in lockup thinking of all I went through to live, only to get to this low point. I decided I had to get back to the kid who, when he was told he wasn't going to make it, said, "No way in hell!" From that point on, I made a commitment to stay sober and turn my life around.

Almost dying saved my life over and over again. I consider myself a survivor of two fatal diseases—cancer and addiction. No matter what happens in my life, I'm alive, and therefore, I'm blessed. Without going through leukemia as a kid, I wouldn't look at it that way. I don't think you really understand yourself until you're tested. When the chips are down and you have to fight, you know you have the strength to make it through any situation.

Cincinnati Dreams Come True: www.cincinnatidreams.org

CHAPTER 9

Planting seeds of hope

Ann Fonfa

Age 61
Stage IV breast cancer
Diagnosed 1993 and 1999
West Palm Beach, Florida

On September 12, 2001, I entered St. Vincent's Hospital in Manhattan, which was serving as a trauma center for victims of the terrorist attacks of 9/11. I was visiting my doctor to hear the results of my recent MRI. It was surreal somehow; sitting in the doctor's office as I'd done many times before, while the world around me was in unimaginable chaos.

Then something remarkable happened. The MRI clearly showed I had no cancer.

With all the tragedy, everyone needed to hear good news. So my doctor did something out of the ordinary. She took me out to the waiting room and announced to the crowd of people there, "Here's a woman who is cancer-free!"

I went outside and started to cry because it really hit me that I was okay for the first time in so many years. And meanwhile, I could see a plume of black smoke coming out of the Trade Center. Several people, who must have thought I was crying over the horrible scene, ran up to me saying, "We'll be okay, don't worry; we'll survive."

I was crying because I was living, and everyone else was crying because so many people had died. It was a very poignant experience.

I had waited so long to hear the words, "cancer-free." When I was first diagnosed with breast cancer at age forty-four in January 1993, I was very ill with chemical sensitivity. I was allergic and reacting to everything—fragrance, carpeting and printed material. They gave me rashes, headaches, and dizziness.

My oncologist said the cancer was early-stage and slow growing. He wanted me to start chemo the following week. I told him about the sensitivity, and he said it didn't matter. I replied, "It matters to me. I don't see how I can do chemo."

I left the office and decided not to do chemotherapy. I figured since the cancer was slow growing, and I would likely react severely to it, chemo would do more harm than good. Radiation, I decided, was not an option for me either. The radiation field included the entire heart and left lung and I didn't want to damage them.

After doing some research, I embarked upon my own plan. I had already eliminated meat from my diet but wasn't paying attention to nutrition. So I improved my eating habits, started taking supplements, and did acupuncture to strengthen my immune system.

Less than two years after I was first diagnosed, I went to a surgeon after feeling another suspicious lump. A biopsy showed the lump was cancerous and also there was another lump underneath it. They told me I had multifocal breast cancer.

Over the next few years, I found a total of twenty-five lumps even after three lumpectomies. Finally I had a left mastectomy, followed a year later by a right mastectomy. I continued to research alternative treatment options and travel to conferences around the country.

At one point, I decided to try high-dose vitamin A. Within three weeks, I saw tumor reduction. But while I felt one getting smaller and softer, another one developed. The vitamins seemed to be working with the one tumor, but not the new one.

After getting the first tumor removed, the pathology report showed it changed from low estrogen-progesterone positive to 90 percent positive. I talked to several oncologists at the San Antonio Breast Cancer Symposium who thought it was very possible that vitamin A could change tumors this way. But when I asked them why no one was using vitamin A, there was no answer. I think many physicians are afraid of vitamins.

I didn't believe strongly in the body-mind connection until I looked back at how things worked for me. When I was diagnosed in 1993, I didn't know anyone with breast cancer. Back then, breast cancer was not discussed as openly as it is today. My first thought was I had such a terrible disease that I was going to die in about five minutes. I spent the weekend comforting my partner, secretly thinking, "This is it."

Sunday night before my surgery, I received a call from a woman I didn't know who told me, "I'm a ten-year survivor." When I heard that, I thought "If she could live ten years, I can, too." My whole being lightened.

When I woke up from my surgery, a nurse said, "You had a lumpectomy, and now you're fine." For years, I'd repeat that to myself and pretty soon, I started believing it.

There has been a lot of research in psychoimmunology, the study of the mind and its effect on the immune system. If you read a sign every morning that says, "I'm great. I'm going to live a long time," it can become a part of your life. Every cell in your body responds to your brain. So you want to think thoughts that are positive and powerful.

Around 1998 two oncologists told me that since the cancer had spread to the chest wall, it was considered stage IV. I told them, "That's absurd, I don't have stage IV!" I never thought my life was in danger; I thought they were wrong.

More determined than ever, I continued to expand my research. I met a Chinese herbalist who had heard about my work and offered to help me. It took me a while to agree to try it because I was worried about how my body would react. I finally took the herbs, then developed hives on every inch of my body.

I later found out the hives were an immune reaction. My entire immune system took a big jolt. But within three days, my chemical sensitivity was reduced by 65 percent. I became so much healthier than I'd ever been before!

My experience fueled my desire to share what I've learned with others. A cancer organization, CancerCare, Inc., found out about my research and asked me to present at their annual conference. I did an outline for the speech and had so much information that I expanded it to a sixty-three page handout.

When I went to the 1997 National Breast Cancer Coalition's Advocacy Training Conference, I brought a hundred copies of it. I was wheeling them around in a hand cart because 6,300 pages were heavy! I tried to give one to each of the fifty states' representatives, so they could bring the information back home. The next year I brought more.

In 1999, I started the Annie Appleseed Project. The name came after brainstorming with my witty mother and poet/writer sister. I went to bed and realized, like Johnnie Appleseed, my aim was to sow seeds of information.

When I launched the Web site, it had twenty-five pages; today it has more than eight thousand. Our volunteers gather information by sending advocates to medical and scientific meetings all over the country. I read journals and abstracts and obtain data from researchers worldwide to put on the site. For the past three years, we've held an annual conference here in Florida, which attracts more than 250 attendees each year. I do all of this as a volunteer. My long-suffering partner, who jokingly refers to himself as Mr. Appleseed, has been supporting me financially and emotionally all along.

People can go to our site and make informed choices. If they still do exactly what the doctor recommended, at least they made a decision based on information rather than fear. We want survivors to have strength and see possibilities that can extend their lives—especially with metastatic disease.

When people describe their success, it's rare that two people have followed the same exact protocols. We don't advise people about what to do because, frankly, we don't have the answers. I just know there are things that work, and if it worked before, maybe it will work again. We now know that everyone is different and a personal approach works, but we don't know yet how to truly personalize care.

One of the things I like least about the medical establishment is when a doctor says, "You have two months to live." Someone just called to tell me her doctor said that. I told her, "They can't know absolutely, so don't believe it. Don't accept it. Spit on it! Stomp on it! They're wrong."

I feel my own experience is proof that doctors can be wrong. My odds should have been terrible with a stage IV diagnosis, yet I've had no evidence of disease since 2001.

The body-mind connection is real. If you have a positive attitude today, that's a better day. Right from the beginning, you're creating happiness while you're on this earth—and no one knows how long that will be.

People used to call me and say, "I'm dying from cancer." I'd say, "Wait, let's have an attitude adjustment. You're *living* with cancer. Get that dying stuff out of your mind."

You may not be hurting yourself in terms of the cancer by not being happy, but you're wasting that day. A cancer researcher from New York walked out of the hospital one day and got hit by a truck. She died at fifty-six. It's what people say in support groups, "You could go out and be hit by a truck." But what if she went around saying, "Oh no, I'm going to die at fifty-six"? What would her life have been like? It's all how you look at it, not what is happening.

The big thing for me is to be able to help people in a meaningful way. I have that joy in my life every day. Making a difference in people's lives; that's what keeps me going. It's an incredible feeling.

The Annie Appleseed Project: www.annieappleseedproject.org
CancerCare Inc.: www.cancercare.org
National Breast Cancer Coalition: www.stopbreastcancer.org
San Antonio Breast Cancer Symposium: www.sabcs.org

CHAPTER 10

Cancer is a disease of love

Evan Mattingly

Age 43
Stage IV neuroendrocrine cancer
Diagnosed 2007
Salt Lake City, Utah

In 2007, a house builder scammed us, and we lost our house and about $100,000 in equity. I thought it was the end of the world. In the middle of our financial crisis, I was diagnosed with a rare form of cancer called neuroendocrin carcinoid cancer.

One oncologist said I had three to five years to live; another said five to eight. I thought, "They're both liars; I'm going to live longer than that!"

I don't ask for trials in my life, but I'm grateful for them because they have made me a stronger person. I never said, "God gave me cancer, and it's going to take me." From the beginning I was determined to fight it. I had a wonderful wife, a teenage son, and a daughter and son-in-law with a baby on the way, so I wanted to stick around.

Like most people in Salt Lake City, I'm a Mormon, and I believe the power of God can heal. We pray for that all the time. With the Lord, anything's possible.

They did the surgery to remove the main tumor, a third of my pancreas, twenty-nine lymph nodes, the gallbladder, and three feet of duodenum, which is the first section of small intestine beneath the stomach. It was radical surgery, which took ten hours. Basically, they had to rebuild my digestive track and reroute it from the stomach.

I didn't eat for five weeks; they fed me intravenously through a PICC line, a tube that's inserted into the large blood vessel leading to the heart. In this way, I could receive nutrition without having it go through my stomach.

After my surgery, my doctor told me I was clear of cancer. Six months later, I had a CT scan, which showed some tumors in my liver. So I had a new treatment called TheraSphere® Radiation in which they inject microscopic radioactive glass beads near the tumors. I've done the procedure three times, most recently last month because more tumors came back and some lymph nodes grew larger. The lymph nodes were along my spine, so they used traditional radiation to treat those.

At my last CT scan, the doctor said, "Everything looks good; your lymph nodes have shrunk down; your liver is clean. Go home and we'll see you in three months." If something else comes up, we'll fight it then. If nothing comes up, I'll go back in three more months.

I feel fantastic right now. I go to work every day, and it's just something I deal with. I'm going to be around for a long time; there's no panic mode. It's life as usual.

I lost about fifty pounds in the year following my surgery. But I was slightly overweight, so I was glad about that. Now I'm at a perfect weight, and my doctors said not to lose any more. Everyone else is trying to lose weight, and I'm trying to keep it on!

I like to joke and have fun; I'm not one to walk around feeling sorry for myself. Early on in my treatment, I walked into my oncologist's office and looked somberly at the three gals sitting at the front desk.

"Hey they just told me I have terminal cancer and have three to five years to live," I said. They just looked at me with big, sad eyes.

"But the good news is…" I continued, "I just lowered my cholesterol!" They all laughed.

Every time I had to go in for a radiation treatment, the techs would say, "Oh good, Evan's here today! Tell us a joke!" After my treatment, I'd sit and shoot the breeze with them for ten minutes and get them laughing. They knew that every time I came in, I'd make them laugh, so they looked forward to it.

People ask, "How can you be so positive all the time?" I answer I could not have dealt with all of this without having good family and friends. I've been pulled up from the depths so many times by the people I love. It just makes me an optimistic person. I don't live in fear or pity.

My wife Julie and I have known each other forever. We both grew up in Salt Lake and were in the same fourth grade class. Julie and I got married when I was twenty-one and she was twenty; we're coming up on our twenty-second anniversary. We know a lot of the same people and both come from large families who all live here in Salt Lake. Everyone has been very supportive.

We just hosted a get-together and invited fifty couples. We had it at our church because it was the only place we knew of that would hold a hundred people. Only one of the invitees couldn't come. We expected at least half couldn't make it. I didn't even tell guests the details; I just said it was going to be a night to remember. They all wanted to be there because they support and love us and want to do what they can to help. Ironically, it had nothing to do with cancer. I just wanted to have a celebration with some entertainment and food to enjoy. We had a fabulous time!

My employer also has been very good to me. They told me whatever time I need, take off; don't worry about it. I received 100 percent of my pay when I had five weeks off for my surgery. This year, some people from work are going to coordinate a fundraising effort for me.

A friend once told me, "Cancer is the disease of love." I asked, "How in the world can that make sense?"

She answered, "Because if you get in a car accident and die, you never have a chance to turn your life around or tell people in your life you love them. But if you get cancer, it's like a warning that you'd better make some changes in your life. You tend to tell people you love them more often and become more compassionate. It's almost like a gift."

My mom died of lung cancer eighteen years ago. She was one of the most loving people in the world. It was hard to see her go through that, but what an opportunity she had to share the love she had for all of us!

Before she died, she sat down and typed a letter to each of her children, knowing she didn't have much time left. She put them in sealed envelopes and gave them to my dad saying, "When I'm gone, I want you to give these to each of the kids." In her letter, she expressed how much she loved me, my family and the Lord. I've taken this to heart and never miss the opportunity to tell people in my life I love them. So, I'm blessed.

That doesn't mean I'm going anywhere soon. I want to spend more time to travel with my family. We love to camp and are planning our first trip for the summer. I love to get out and ride my motorcycle in the mountains and plan to do more of that. I have a goal to go on a cruise and drive the Redwood Forest in California someday. I'm looking forward to a really good summer and to many more summers to come.

After my first surgery, I told my doctors it was my first birthday. The next year, it was my second birthday. This coming year, it will be my third birthday. I plan on having a lot more birthdays.

Attitude

Discussion Questions

1. Looking at the stories in this book, how did the individuals' attitudes help them?

2. Much has been said about the body-mind connection. Could having a positive attitude help promote healing? Have you found this to be true in your personal experience?

3. Some argue that being pressured to have a positive attitude can be detrimental. What are your thoughts on this?

4. How do you balance being positive with feeling "less positive" emotions such as fear, sadness, and anger?

5. Brenda Michaels and Evan Mattingly talk about "finding the gift in cancer." What gifts have you realized as a result of your or a loved one's diagnosis?

Part III

Support

CHAPTER 11

A mother's love

Rose Paul

Age 49
Choriocarcinoma
Diagnosed 1982
Charleston, South Carolina

In October 1982, I was twenty-one years old and had been married not quite a year. I'd delivered my son Jason three months before, but I'd never stopped bleeding. My doctor knew something was wrong and sent me to a gynecologic-oncologist. He told me I had choriocarcinoma, cancer of the uterine lining.

I remember sitting outside the X-ray department. Through the open door, I heard the radiologist call the doctor saying, "She has metastases in both lungs." He could have been talking about anybody, but I knew it was me.

This is a very aggressive cancer, and back in 1982, there wasn't much hope for survival. There were only two hospitals on the East Coast that would even touch me. My doctor was the only one who knew anything about the disease. He said, "I had one other patient with this kind of cancer, and we lost her. At the rate this is growing and how aggressive it is, I can't promise you'll be here for Christmas."

He wanted me to check into the hospital that day to start treatment. I told him, "I can't do that; I have a three-month-old son! Who's going to take care of him?" He put it plainly to me, emphasizing that I wouldn't be around to see my baby's first tooth if I didn't get treatment. I said, "Okay, I'll be there in the morning."

My mother took care of my son while I was in the hospital. I did radiation and aggressive chemo. I'd been in the hospital one week when my husband was visiting. I stood up to get something from the bedside table. He said, "Rose, sit down!" Underneath me was a pool of blood. I had started to hemorrhage.

I had emergency surgery to remove my uterus. The next day, I woke up and found my mother holding my hand and crying. I reached down to my stomach, felt the bandage and started crying. I'd always wanted more children.

My mom said, "It's all right honey; your son is here, and he's healthy. What's important is seeing him grow up. It's going to be rough, but I know you're a fighter and you don't like to quit. You need to fight with everything you have." She made me promise, and I did.

My mom had quite a way of motivating me. Another time when I was very sick, my family was called to my bedside. When I opened my eyes, she said, "I shed my last tear over you, young lady. You're getting better right now because I won't stand over the grave of my child!"

With an Irish mother, you listen or else, so I listened to her. I knew I couldn't do that to her. I would joke that if I did die, she would probably kill me.

I'd always say, "I'm going to beat this because I want to see Jason grow up." I stayed in the hospital five months and missed him terribly. I wanted to put my arms around my baby, and I couldn't. I was allowed to visit him in the lobby when my mom brought him. Sometimes when I was in isolation, I couldn't even see him. It hurt to know other people were raising my child. I had to square with that.

The chemo eliminated the cancer in my lungs, and I was released from the hospital. When I came home, my son was eight months old. I held on to him for dear life, carrying him everywhere I went. I held him when he was sleeping and would just look at him. I was so happy to see Jason again. People said I was going to spoil that child, but I didn't care. For five months, I couldn't carry him at all. I was making up for lost time.

I had a blood test every week. Eventually it tapered down to every month, then every three months, and six months. Finally, they said I was essentially cured. In June 1983, I was given my permanent walking papers.

But things were not so positive in my personal life. My son wasn't a year old yet when my husband told me he wanted a divorce. He blamed the cancer for the breakup, saying it put too much stress on him. My mother, in her forthright way, reassured me that our breakup was a good thing because, "If you have a pimple, you want to get rid of it early before it gets worse."

That made sense to me. I stopped blaming myself for being sick because it wasn't my fault. I told my mother, "You are moving to Florida next year; I think I'll go with you." So I bundled up my baby, and we hit the road for Florida.

In hindsight, I think it was meant to be. If I hadn't left, I wouldn't have met my second husband, Jeff. We were working at the same company, where I did drafting work. For four months, he kept asking me to dinner but I refused because I was afraid of getting burned again. He finally wore me down.

That was twenty-three years ago, and we've been together like bread and butter ever since. I find it odd that my husband's birthday is April 21, the same day I was released from the hospital. Call it luck; I know fortune smiled on me—when I walked out of the hospital and when Jeff walked into my life.

I didn't know back then how much Jeff would mean to me. The cancer was gone, but the damage was done without our knowing it. In 1997, I started to get really bad back pains that wouldn't go away. I went to the doctor who told me I had severe wear on my spine. I learned my bone density was very thin, not good for someone who was relatively young and in good health. They later determined it was because of all of my radiation treatments and scans.

Year after year, my back keeps getting worse. I deal with chronic pain, so I have a morphine implant that helps me get through my days. But when you come right down to it, I'm alive. I've had the chance to see my son grow up into a fine young man and have had a good life with my husband. I'm very happy.

Jeff and I have been through everything together. He's my soul mate. Jeff tells me, "I don't care if you don't do housework at all; I know how to vacuum and do wash." He comes home for lunch to make sure I'm okay. I'm unable to stand and cook, so he cooks for me. I have difficulty eating sometimes; food will taste metallic because of the morphine. So he'll make me something I like from scratch because he knows I'll eat it. This guy never cooked before in his life before we got married!

I beat myself up sometimes because he works all day as a computer tech then comes home and works, too. I try to help out, but he tells me, "Go lie down. You're going through a rough patch. I'll take care of it." When he's not working, he insists we go out and get some sunshine. He'll put me in my wheelchair, and we'll do one of the touristy things around here.

I can't work because I'm unable to stand or sit very long. But I do a lot of volunteer work with the American Cancer Society as a patient advocate and helping with the Relay for Life, among other things. I enjoy giving back because they did so much for my family when I was sick.

It helps me too. So many times, I see patients who look like they've been hit in the face with a fish. I talked to a gentleman who was just diagnosed with prostate cancer. He said, "I guess I should write a will now." I told him, "A will is the last thing to worry about now; we need to get you treatment. Prostate cancer can be healed." After talking with me, he didn't feel like his end was near anymore.

Jeff gets mad at me sometimes because he thinks I am too personally involved. He's afraid one of my patients will die, and I won't be able to take it. I don't worry about that because I think, "We're going to win. We're going to beat it."

I have so much to be grateful for. My husband and I may not be up in the mountains hiking, but we have a very good life. Some days I struggle, and some days I'm fine. But at least I don't have my life on the line anymore. I'm happy I got see my son graduate and get married. They just had a daughter, Emily Rose. He's going to be a great dad, but I'm going to be a fantastic grandma! This time around, I'm not missing out on showering love onto a little child.

American Cancer Society: Relay for Life: www.relayforlife.org

CHAPTER 12

Blessings and blooms

Susan Farmer

Age 49
Stage IV breast cancer
Diagnosed 1994, 2001, and 2005
Boston, Massachusetts

I sit on my bench and look at my lovely garden. It's filled with blue hydrangea, holly bushes, salvia, roses, and other colorful plants and flowers. There's beautiful wildlife, too. Even though I live in the city, rabbits and birds come and feed in my yard. It sounds like a scene from Cinderella, but they all flock around me. It makes me feel really connected with nature.

I'm a very nurturing person, and the biggest heartache of my life was my inability to have children. Having a garden gives me something to love and nurture. I love the garden and it loves me back with continuous blooms, year after year.

I was thirty-four when I was first diagnosed with breast cancer. My tumor was very small, so doctors recommended a lumpectomy and radiation. I didn't do chemo. Many people in my situation would have agreed to it, but my husband and I had a strong desire to have children and were trying to get pregnant at the time. I also had the complication of Type 1 diabetes.

After my first diagnosis, I went seven years without cancer. I honestly thought it was behind me. But it returned. I had a mastectomy, but still no chemo. My oncologist was concerned about potential complications due to diabetes. She presented my case to a board of oncologists from three hospitals. Half recommended chemo and the other half recommended hormonal treatments. I chose the latter.

I did well for a while on hormonal treatments, and then the cancer would return again and again. Finally, I had no choice but to do chemo. I endured eleven rounds and actually did fairly well. But it did worsen the condition of my already damaged nervous system. I still have residual problems because of it.

Four months after my final chemo, the cancer returned. This time, they found it on the other side of my body in the lymphatic system, which was considered stage IV cancer.

My oncologist had seen a study of women who had both their cancerous and healthy breasts removed. While they found no cancer in the healthy breast, in 10 percent of the women, they did find it in the lymphatic channel above the healthy breast. They concluded that in a very small number of women, the cancer found in the other side may be the primary cancer. My doctor therefore concluded the cancer found in my lymph nodes might be where the cancer originated; not a metastasis. She told me, if this were the case, there was the potential for a "cure." I hung on to that idea for dear life.

Because of the aggressive nature of the cancer, she proposed a radical procedure: removing a few ribs so they could go in deep and excise the cancerous tissue; then performing skin and muscle grafts to close the wound. I went to several other hospitals for additional doctors' opinions. They were concerned the wound wouldn't close because of my diabetes and wondered why I would be put through such a procedure, since stage IV is incurable.

I wondered why my oncologist would be the "Lone Ranger" in her plan of action and decided to ask her. She explained that, since I went to research hospitals for second opinions, its doctors were beholden to research grant protocols. She, however, worked for a hospital that allows their physicians to think outside the box.

But I really held on to what she said next: "Every patient deserves to be thought of as the person who could be that one in a million. Therefore, I propose attacking your cancer with both barrels loaded. I could be wrong, but then again, I could be right."

I agreed to the surgery and spent ten days in the hospital and three months recuperating at my home. It was nothing short of a miracle that the wound closed.

The biggest miracle of all, though, was that the surgery worked! Subsequent scans showed no evidence of disease. It's been three years, and I've had clear scans ever since.

I think it's important to have a team like mine that's willing to keep trying. If there's any chance a treatment can extend your life, you owe it to yourself and those who love you to try. My doctor also says, "Just hang on! We're so close to finding a cure we can almost taste it." I think that's a very good message to give patients.

At a recent oncologist's visit, a new nurse who never met me before said, "You've been cancer-free for three years; that's amazing!" I looked at her and my doctor and said "Yes, I am a miracle!" My doctor agreed and said, "Sure, you never give credit to science!" We all laughed.

I'm a spiritual person and a Christian; I pray to God. I believe that God is the author of miracles. I also believe that God is the author of the scientific part of such good news. It seems when people believe, it causes the body to relax. I think it's really crucial to your health and well-being. Stress can only destroy the body. A positive, relaxed outlook is very healing. My spiritual beliefs play a huge role in my current state of health.

The other major thing that helped me was the ability to give and receive love. I have very beautiful people in my life who think about those little things that mean so much and give life richness. I am very blessed to have a wonderful husband who hugs me when I need to be hugged; I don't have to tell him. He never fails me when it comes to supporting my emotional health in regard to my medical problems.

It must have been exhausting for him to have a wife with one medical crisis after another from the very beginning of our relationship. Yet he has never made me feel bad for having burdened him— he doesn't consider me a burden. He adores me, and this is the most healing of all.

I also have a wonderful mom, who at eighty-four years young, still watches over me. I have three siblings and one, who lives nearby, calls me every single day to check on me. I don't know what I would do without her calls. She's my lifeline, and I can always count on her to be there if I need her. My other two other siblings live further away, but are also there when I need them. My nieces and nephews mean the absolute world to me. I love them as if they were my own children; they add so much light and love to my life.

And finally, I have an amazing group of supportive friends. Most of my friends work in social services, so they have an altruistic nature. They give and give and give some more. I have many friends who continuously call to check on me, even in my times of remission, when I need less.

There were times during these last few years when I had been so sick, I couldn't even walk, go outside or receive visitors. I am a very social person and not being able to see people was the hardest part of all.

When I was recovering from my chest wall resection, depression was beginning to creep in. It was a long winter in New England, and the world was dark and gray. I knew I needed something to keep me going, add color to my world, and make me feel alive. So I began searching for cancer organizations that could help me.

I have always loved to garden, but didn't know how to landscape so it would look artistic. I thought, "There has to be a gardening program for cancer patients." I discovered Hope in Bloom, a nonprofit organization that plants gardens free of charge at the homes of Massachusetts residents undergoing breast cancer treatment.

When I found their Web site, I started crying with joy. The founder Roberta Hershon formed the organization after she lost her best friend

Beverly to breast cancer. Roberta was inspired to start the organization by what she did for Beverly during treatment: taking care of Beverly's garden and keeping her house filled with flowers.

The Hope in Bloom director came to my house along with a landscape designer. They were so loving and sincere in wanting to give me this gift. My husband and I had the opportunity to give input, and they followed our suggestions exactly. They respected what we both wanted and how much upkeep we would be able to do.

I happened to be one of the first people to benefit from the program. I was having a very hard time preparing for this experience. It was so uncomfortable receiving help. Since I worked in social services, my life's work has always been about giving to others. I had never been on the receiving end, so my friends actually had to talk me into accepting the garden.

On the day of the garden installation, an army of volunteers appeared at my door. The youngest was in high school and the oldest in her seventies. The volunteers all greeted me with smiles and hugs. Their sincerity was amazing! I was finally able to relax and receive this wonderful garden after realizing there is a gift in the act of giving, too. They, too, were touched by the experience.

When they finished the garden, it looked exquisite—the garden of dreams! I never imagined it would be so professional and magazine-worthy. My husband and I shed tears, as well as did several of the volunteers. It was a moment I'll never forget.

What's so beautiful is the garden continues to bloom, year after year. And, in a way, it continues to bloom for others. Some of the volunteers were so moved by installing my garden that they decided to plant gardens for other cancer patients. They invited their friends to volunteer, who also enlisted their friends. This garden is the gift that keeps on giving.

A garden is like a relationship: the more seeds you sow, the more you get back. Spend your life sowing love, and it will bloom over and over, continuously giving you blessing upon blessing throughout your life. I have received so many blessings, and for that, I am grateful.

Hope in Bloom: www.hopeinbloom.org

CHAPTER 13

With a little help from my friends

Steve Scott

Age 48
Stage IV colon cancer
Diagnosed 2004
Cincinnati, Ohio

"Screw it. I'm going to have fun for a year and half and then they can bury me."

That's almost what I said when I was diagnosed with stage IV colon cancer. If it hadn't been for my wife Cassandra, there wouldn't have been a decision to make. I would have gone out with a bang and wouldn't have done chemo. But it was a new marriage and we were trying to have kids.

My life had been a dream. Maybe that's why I didn't get married until I was forty. I used to be fearless. I rode a motorcycle, flew planes, and scuba dived. I thought, "I had a good life, so I'm ready to die." But then I realized, "I have this wonderful woman now. You never know; I could duplicate the first half of my life with the second half."

I was playing drums in my band the night before Valentine's Day 2004, when I felt this cramp that did not go away. I stayed awake all night. Cassandra took me to the emergency room first thing in the morning. They did an ultrasound and told me I had spots covering the entire liver. A needle biopsy confirmed it was colon cancer that had spread to the lymph nodes and liver.

We didn't know about stages of cancer. We thought, "This is going to be ugly for the next couple of years and then we can move on." Then we really got hit. The next week, Cassandra, my sister, and I went to my doctor's office and found out it was one of the worst kind of cancers, and we were at the last stage of it.

"You're not a candidate for surgery, and I wouldn't advise chemo," he told us. "I would probably just enjoy my life. You have about eighteen months to live. The chemo would probably only prolong your life a couple of months. But the pain you'd get from it would decrease the quality of your life so much; there would be no sense in doing it."

We just started bawling. It was bad enough that just a week before, we heard I had cancer; but then we got the news that it was terminal. We sat on the couch and cried for days. I called work immediately and told them I needed some time to figure this out. They told me to take as much time as I needed. My wife did the same.

We thought, "Why us?" We couldn't imagine how this could happen to two people who were pretty nice. That's when I stopped believing in God and said, "This isn't right. I didn't deserve this."

I had no hope that I would make it past eighteen months. I went to five oncologists in three different cities who told me the same thing: I was going to die. At that point, I decided to do some research because I didn't know anything about cancer. I found a surgeon at Memorial Sloan-Kettering Cancer Center in New York City who was one of the leading experts on colon cancer that spread to the liver.

I faxed him seventeen pages of medical records and asked if he'd take me as a patient. His office told me, "You have an appointment next Monday at 4 P.M. Be there." That was the beginning.

He told me, "We're not going to kid you; you're in bad shape. But we have a lot of experience with patients like you and we think there is something we can do." They didn't shut the door like everyone else did. They gave me a little grain of hope.

So every month, we would fly up to New York to get scans and chemo. In three years, I received a total of fifty-seven chemo treatments and five surgeries. Because I was young and strong, I was on very high dose chemo. They gave me twice the amount they gave other people.

There were several things that got me through the rounds of chemo. People told me I could heal myself and to try the alternative methods first. I said, "There's no way I'm going to do that. I'm going to let the doctors do it. But I'll try to supplement the medical treatments with other things." It made me feel like I was covering all the bases. I figured, if you're going to beat the unbeatable, you better pull every arrow out of the bucket. And I did.

I had healing touch weekly and talked to a shrink every two weeks. One of the best things I ever did was go to the Wellness Community's support group. My wife went to the group for caregivers. We met so many people there. You can talk to friends or relatives all you want, but they aren't in the same orbit. You need to talk with others who are going through it. I learned very early on not to try to tackle this by myself. There's strength in numbers.

I saw other people going through this, and found there was something I could learn from each one of them. There was a nun in her late sixties in my group who received eighteen heavy chemo treatments. She was talking about it like she was taking candy. She was so tough and somehow was thriving. There was another guy on a chemo regimen similar to mine who played racquetball the day he came home from chemo. He was ten years older than me. I listened to how they accomplished this and said, "That's what I need to do."

Cassandra was thirty-four when I was diagnosed. She was very young to get this diagnosis. She was a model then, doing commercials and advertisements around town. Cassandra was like I was; she was a real tough cookie who didn't talk with or need help from anyone. To someone like that, cancer is a death sentence. But she realized, with our situation, she needed all the help she could get.

By going to support groups, she saw extraordinary things other spouses were experiencing. This helped her to reach out, which was very helpful to her and to our relationship.

I was lucky to have several great people in my life. My sister was a jewel; an unbelievable help. She took two weeks off from work and came here immediately. She went back and forth from Virginia Beach for doctor appointments, chemo sessions, and for all the surgeries.

I also had two good friends: Rich, my tennis partner, and Jeff, who played music with me in a band. Both were really integral to my success. When I "had no gasoline in the tank," Rich would make me play tennis with him because he knew it's what I needed to get through my next round of chemo. He'd send me emails, saying "I can't play tennis without you. You're my partner. If you don't play, I don't play." He did this week after week for two years.

Jeff sat with me during my chemo sessions. It was unbelievable; a married guy my age would come over and baby-sit me during my chemo rounds!

Finally my treatments ended and I was told my cancer was gone. You'd think I'd be elated, but I was in sheer depression for more than a year afterwards. I kept saying, "Now what?" You spend so many years just hanging on, then all of sudden; they tell you you're disease-free.

Cancer has definitely taken a toll on my life, but it has given me a lot too. I'm a recovering drug addict. I did a lot of coke as a kid, and stopped twenty-one years ago. I prayed for years to get back in touch with myself emotionally because I was a cold fish kind of guy. When you are using, you kind of go on automatic pilot and cut off your emotions. So when you stop using drugs and alcohol, you're left with an empty house.

I feel things really deeply now, good or bad. I like that. I want to feel. Little did I know that it would take cancer to get back my emotions.

I'm mending my relationship with God. I absolutely believe there is a Higher Power, but I have trouble with the Christian version of it. I read spiritual books, but now I'm uncomfortable with the church setting. I keep trying to get back into going to church.

Cassandra and I have our struggles, but we're doing much better with our communication, thanks to some counseling. Our love couldn't be any deeper, and our relationship is better today than it was before the cancer. We've seen the edge of the abyss, so there's not much now that can really make us think, "This life sucks." We know what sucks, and that was cancer.

Another thing that changed is that both of us know we need to make a difference in the world. We understand now material things aren't what we need in life. Connections to other people, empathy, and helping others are what's important.

I give back now by volunteering at the Wellness Community, working at the front desk and helping with fundraising. I was national sales manager at a meat company. I didn't fit in my career; I loved the money, but it wasn't for me. Right now I'm struggling with what I want to do. I'm trying to enjoy every day, have fun, and not plan too far in the future.

Cassandra was in retail. Now she has a job at a community college helping underprivileged, young people get into school and make it in the world, just as she did herself. She was the first person in her family to go to college. She has that story to tell.

My advice to people who are going through a similar diagnosis is to never let a doctor take your hope away. I think about when I was diagnosed with cancer, someone was smart enough to send me Lance Armstrong's book. That's all I needed to give me hope.

I have been cancer-free for three years and I'm having the chance to make my second half of my life even better than the first. I have good friends, a wonderful marriage, and the opportunity to give hope to others. I'm a lucky, lucky guy.

The Cancer Support Community—The Wellness Community and Gilda's Club: www.cancersupportcommunity.org

Photo Section

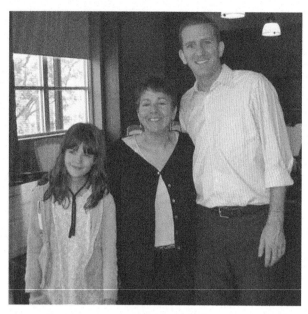

(Left to right) Chrissy and Tami Boehmer visit Doug Ulman, CEO and president of the Lance Armstrong Foundation, at the LIVESTRONG headquarters in Austin.

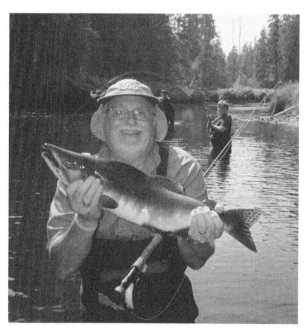

Greg Barnhill shows off his big catch and zest for life during a trip to Alaska.

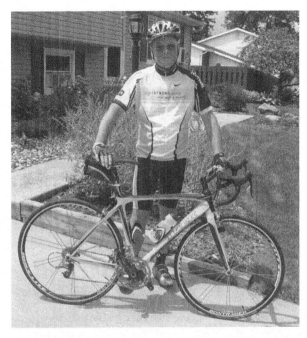

Jack Gray uses his bike to raise cancer funds, awareness, and hope.

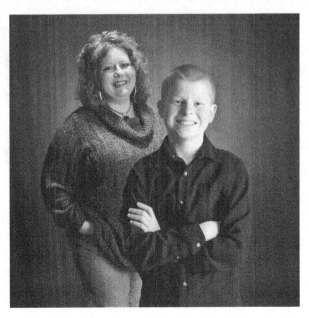

Diagnosed with ovarian cancer while pregnant with her son Johnathan,
Cathy Wolfe fought to save both their lives.

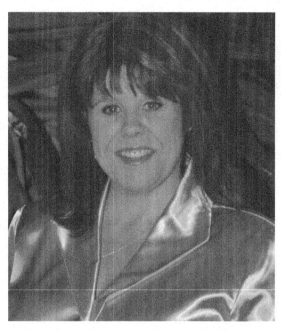

*Penny Feddick leads the way for LIVESTRONG in
Arizona as she seeks funding for cancer research.*

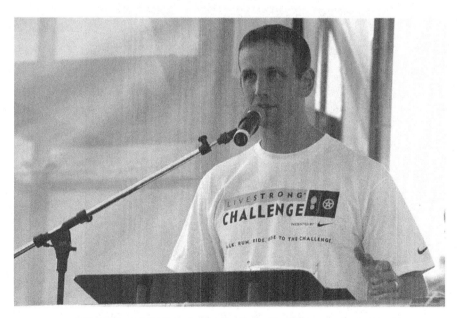

*Bob Kiesendahl beat leukemia and tells of his experience at
fundraising events, such as this one for LIVESTRONG.*

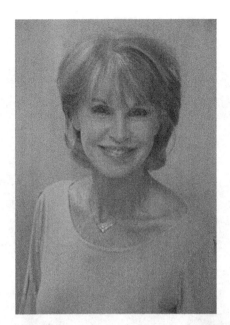

Brenda Michaels experienced a spiritual transformation while healing her cancer.

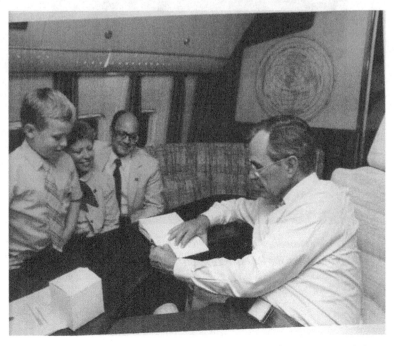

Paul Falk's scrapbook includes this photo of his ride on Air Force Two with his parents Lisa and Ken Weber and Vice President George H. W. Bush (circa 1987).

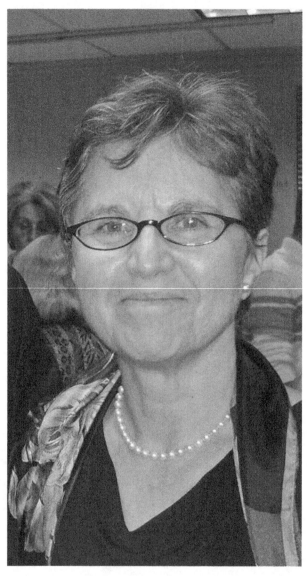

Ann Fonfa triumphed over cancer with integrative methods. She now shares what she learns through the Annie Appleseed Project.

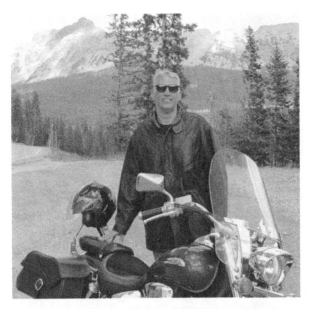

Evan Mattingly loves riding his motorcycle through the mountains as a way to celebrate living.

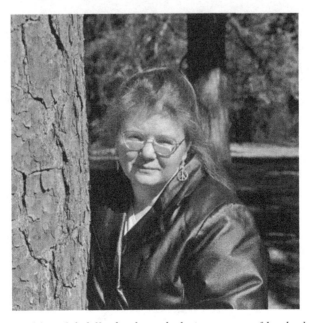

Rose Paul lives life fully thanks to the loving support of her husband.

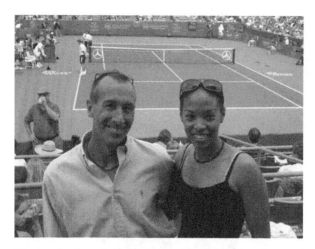

Steve and Cassandra Scott enjoy many activities now that Steve is cancer-free, including this ATP Tennis Tournament in Cincinnati.

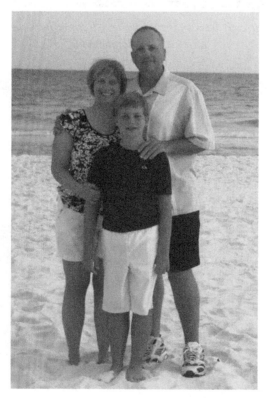

Christine Dittmann, with her son Drake and husband Steve, survived both Hurricane Katrina and cancer with courage, humor, and grace.

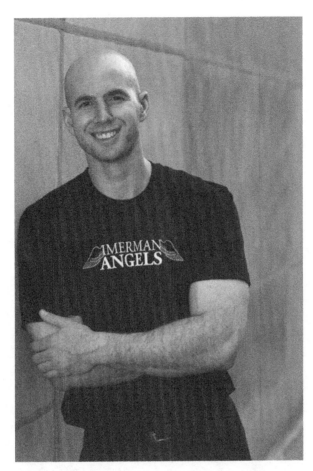

Jonny Imerman wears his T-shirt everywhere he goes to promote his cancer mentorship organization.

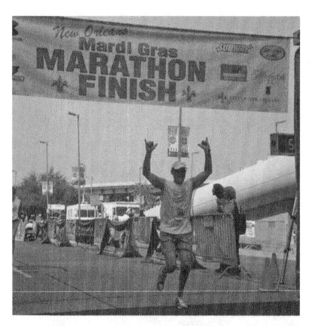

Twenty-three years after being told he had six months to live,
Dave Massey competes in marathons like this one.

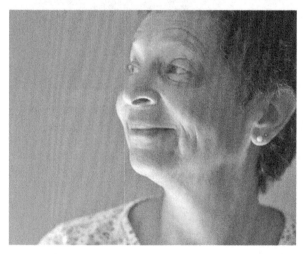

Yvonne Cooper uses her art to express her transformation since cancer.

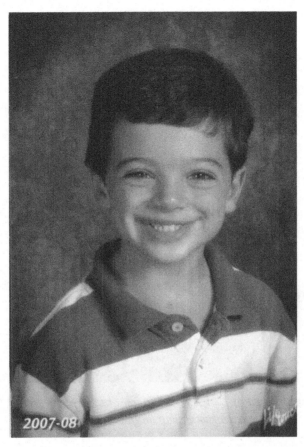

They didn't think Charlie Capodanno would live six months when he was diagnosed as a baby with brain and spinal cancer. This school picture shows they were wrong.

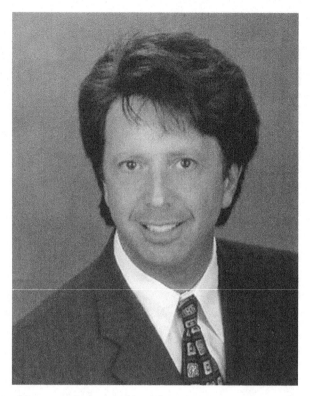

Daniel Levy took charge of his life and cancer treatment when he was diagnosed with brain cancer in 1991.

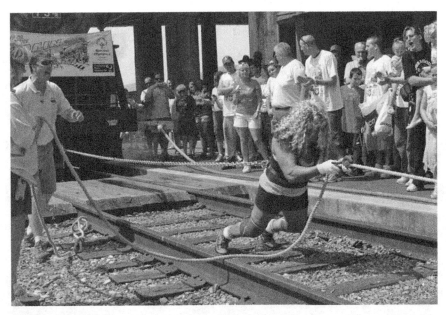

Strong Woman and cancer survivor Mary Jacobson pulls a 250-ton train for charity.

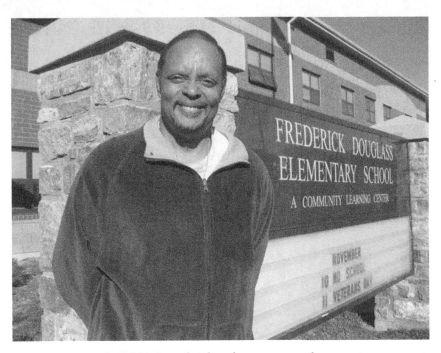

*Buzz Sheffield believes he's here for a reason, such as tutoring
kids at this inner-city school.*

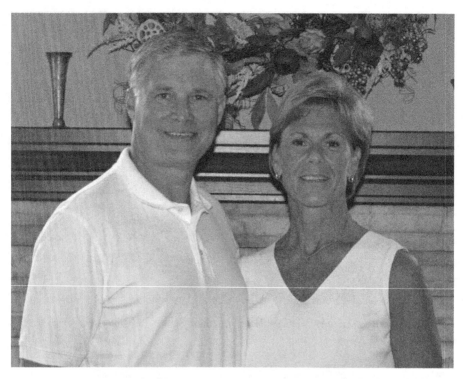

Denny and Theresa Seewer credit God's grace for Denny's
thirty-five years of cancer-free survival.

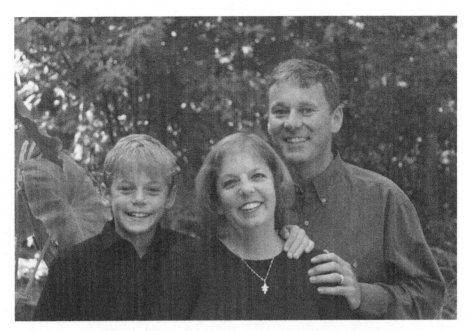

Kathy Wood, picture here with her son Jarrett and husband Brian, is spreading her message of hope through her online ministry.

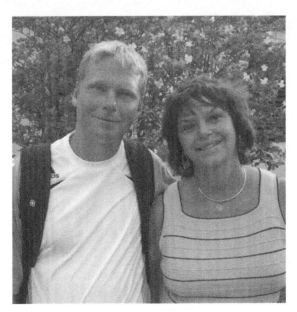

Nancy Hamm, pictured with her son Keith, has found new meaning in her life since her cancer diagnosis.

CHAPTER 14

Hurricanes, humor, and healing

Christine Dittmann

Age 43
Thyroid cancer and stage IV ovarian cancer
Diagnosed in 2005
Baton Rouge, Louisiana

We lived about ten minutes east of the French Quarter, six blocks from the Mississippi River. I had an appointment to see an oncologist the Monday Hurricane Katrina hit. Just days before, I learned I had another storm brewing.

The previous month, I successfully recovered from thyroid cancer surgery, as well as a repair to an abdominal hernia. Because of its high survival rates, they told me, "If you have cancer, thyroid is the one to have." I knew I would have to have a radioactive iodine treatment in order to completely treat the cancer, but I wasn't worried. I thought I was out of the woods.

But soon I started to feel cramped and bloated. Over four days, my stomach grew bigger and bigger until I looked nine months pregnant.

I thought I might have been allergic to the mesh they used in the hernia repair. I was having trouble walking and breathing, so I had an ultrasound. They found two and a half liters of fluid in my abdomen! I felt so much better after they drained it, but later that night, the fluid came back completely. It sounded like a faucet had been turned on.

The Thursday before the storm, the doctors performed a CT scan and a biopsy. It was ovarian cancer. This would be the eye of the storm, the one I had always dreaded.

I couldn't believe it. Eighteen months previously, I had a total hysterectomy and prophylactic mastectomy. I had the surgeries after discovering my maternal aunts and I tested positive for the BRCA 1 gene mutation, which significantly increases the risk of breast and ovarian cancer. Ironically, my fraternal twin sister tested negative for the mutation. My mother died of breast cancer; and my maternal grandmother and one of my maternal aunts died of ovarian cancer. Another one of my maternal aunts survived ovarian cancer and has been cancer-free for nine years. It was definitely in my family, and I wanted to do my best to prevent it.

People with the BRCA 1 genetic mutation, however, still have a 1 to 3 percent chance of getting cancer in the remaining tissue if their ovaries are removed. I was part of that small percentage group. It was like winning some strange lottery with an awful prize.

That evening after my scan results, my dad arrived unexpectedly from Michigan to be with me for my first oncology appointment. Like everyone else in the area, we started watching the TV weather closely. My dad went out to buy hurricane supplies just in case.

On Saturday, my husband Steve took me back to the emergency room in order to drain more fluid from my abdomen, as well as my lungs. When we returned home, we saw the TV report announcing the order to evacuate. We had until Sunday morning to leave.

There wasn't much time to gather our belongings. I grabbed our important papers, wedding photos, and my seven-year-old son Drake's baby album. I begged my family to let me stay, saying, "I'm too sick to go. Every time they say there's going to be a big storm, it never happens." But of course, they made me go. Now I know I, like so many others, wouldn't be alive to talk about it if I had stayed.

Sunday morning we piled into two cars to travel to my nephew's home in Baton Rouge. It was only seventy miles away, but it took us seven hours because of all the evacuation traffic. When we finally arrived, we sat glued to the television, watching as the storm hit the Gulf Coast. In a matter of hours, it was over. It didn't look like there was much damage, so we assumed we could return the next day.

When we woke up we had the shock of our lives. The levees had broken and the majority of New Orleans was under water. On TV, we watched the utter chaos at the Convention Center and the Superdome. We saw bodies floating in the water, babies crying for food and water, and some elderly people dead in their wheelchairs. We sat transfixed, watching as water engulfed our neighborhood, completely covering roofs of houses.

Now our plans had to change. I needed to find an oncologist, and soon. Steve's sister Janet called from New Jersey with news she had secured an appointment for me with a top gynecology/oncology physician at the University of Pennsylvania. She invited us to stay with her family. It was never said, but we all knew we would be living there for a long time.

Three days later, I arrived at the airport in New Jersey. I was in a complete daze. I barely remember the flight or the ride to their house in Moorestown. When we arrived, we discovered a large portion of Steve's family had already evacuated there. In all, there were five families, comprised of eighteen people and four dogs living under one roof.

The morning after I arrived, Janet took me to the University of Pennsylvania for testing with one of the top ten doctors in the nation for ovarian cancer, Dr. Stephen Rubin. He told me the cancer had spread to the lungs, lymph nodes, and liver…and it was incurable. In so many words, I was being told I would be fighting this for the rest of my life.

I immediately started chemo and was hospitalized for several days. Friends were just beginning to reach me on my cell phone and some were in tears. I didn't understand why, but later learned they thought we had stayed and were lost in the storm.

Back at Janet's, we tried to keep the kids away from the TV news, but we all saw the wreckage that was left behind. In the area of New Orleans where we lived, St. Bernard Parish, a majority of people stayed. There were a lot of boat rescues, but many people died. It was hard for me because the hospital, where I worked as a public relations specialist, was right smack in that area too. There was no air conditioning. They didn't have enough water. The CEO was the last one to leave after seven days of this.

A week or so later, we got word that residents were allowed to re-turn to the city. So Steve drove the twenty-four hour trip to see the condition of our beloved hundred-year-old home. When he reached the Parish, it looked like a war zone. The National Guard was there, and residents had to show ID to enter.

Steve made his way to the house, and what he saw he will never forget. There were boats on top of houses, houses in the middle of the street, and cars inside houses. When he reached our home, he knew we would never be able to return. Mold had already grown on the walls, the roof had numerous holes, and pieces of the back porch had blown off. The plumbing and electricity were months away from work-ing again. And all of our possessions had either floated away or were destroyed by the storm.

Steve stayed that night at a friend's house in another Parish and then started back to New Jersey. That's when his ten-month fight with the insurance company and my fight with cancer began.

We quickly settled into our new home. Drake started school with his seven-year-old cousin. Within three weeks, family members started to leave Janet's home. If their home had been destroyed, they went to live with other family members.

It was unbelievable how many people helped us. Friends and family raised money for us, including my best friend from high school who started a Web site. My graduating class, 1984, has always been close and they reached out to us when we needed it the most. My dad is a city manager and has lots of friends, so we heard from people all over the country. One of my friends sent me a portable DVD player so I could watch movies while taking chemo.

There was an outpouring of support from people of Moorestown, too. In 2005, *Money* magazine voted Moorestown the best small town to live in America. Based on everything its residents did for us, it certainly delivered on that.

I lost my job and the insurance I received from it. An area philanthropist met with us after reading about us in the paper, and then generously paid our insurance for a while. Since we only packed for three days when we left, people from the fire department and churches dropped clothes and food at our doorstep. The local grocery store donated gift cards. One generous family even donated a beautiful two-bedroom condo for us to use when our family and friends visited. And we had many visitors, including my family and a glorious parade of beloved friends.

Four months after Katrina, we all returned to New Orleans to visit the rest of Steve's family for Christmas. That was the first time Drake and I had been to the house. I couldn't go in because of the environmental hazards; Drake and Steve wore masks and other protective gear. I cried, memories of Drake's first steps running through my head. But it was just a house. The important thing was we were all together and everyone was safe.

We finally received our insurance settlement so Steve went on ahead and looked for a home for us. I only saw three pictures of the house. My sister didn't know how we could buy a house without seeing it first. I told her, you could if you have been living in one room for the past ten months!

I went back to my oncologist in Baton Rouge and had a CT scan, which showed I was clear of cancer. I was off chemo for a month, but the symptoms started again and we found out the cancer had returned. It spread all over the colon, vagina, and bladder. I underwent a five-hour surgery; they had to remove a lot of the colon. After that, they put me on another chemo regimen that most people can only tolerate for six months; I was on it for eighteen. It stopped working after a while, so I started a new chemo. This last PET scan showed it had been shrinking, but some big nodules remained. So I had another surgery. Now I'm back on chemo and once again feeling the breeze on my bare head.

My neighbors here have all been wonderful. When I have surgeries, chemo, or other procedures they cook meals for us or take Drake for the day. I couldn't do it without them.

Drake was seven when I was diagnosed. At first, your instinct is to protect your children so you don't talk about it. When I looked back, that's what my parents did when my mother had cancer—and we were adults. Steve and I went to a counselor, who said, "The more you things you hide from him, the more he is going to interpret and make things up in his head." He suggested being honest, so that's what we started doing. I said, "I have cancer. It doesn't mean I'm going to die. I just have to go to chemo and have surgeries."

I've come to realize cancer is just one part of our lives. Drake handles it very well. He's eleven now and has come to the age when his empathy has developed. He asks, "How did chemo go today. Do you need anything?" One counselor told us that helps make him part of your recovery, so he's not on the outside and can communicate with you.

With the hurricane coming at the same time of my diagnosis, I never had the chance to process what was going on with me. I was so ill, I don't even remember part of the trip to Pennsylvania and the first hospital visit. It took me a long time—really, up until the last six months—to sit down and think about it. I know that sounds funny, but when you're in a survival state, you're just fighting, fighting, fighting. You don't think about what's happened. Now it really hits me hard when I hear about people who are going through treatment or see something on TV about the hurricane.

We have a sense of humor, and that helps. We love funny movies, and all of us are good at laughing at ourselves. Some people might think our humor is kind of dark. I'll say to Steve, "You know I'm dying here," and he'll say, "Well, can you get on with it?" Or when I have a good medical report he'll say, "There goes my Corvette for another three months." He recently went on a diet and is losing weight, so I asked him if he was getting ready for his second wife. He's been married before, and he reminded me that I *am* his second wife.

It also helps to give back. I co-facilitate a support group at the cancer center in New Orleans and write for their newsletter. God gave me the talent to write. I try to help people realize they can still have a full life after they're diagnosed. It may not be what you expected, but you can still be happy. I recently was nominated as a "health care hero" for my volunteer work at a ceremony hosted by the New Orleans business paper.

I feel like I beat the odds so far. I have a different outlook now about God. When I'm feeling so bad that I can't go on anymore, I can feel His arms wrapped around me. It gives me such a feeling of serenity and peace. I can accept whatever happens because I know where I'm going after I die. Hopefully, I'll see my mom and others in my family.

My husband and son are so close. Steve has done such a good job with Drake; I'm not worried about them. But that doesn't mean I will ever stop fighting. I don't really have a choice. A child needs a mother as long as possible. It's my job to raise him and see him have a happy, healthy life. I want him to know that I fought as hard as I could fight.

Everyone in my family says I'm like the bionic woman; I'm so strong. I always say, it's not me. I couldn't have made it without my wonderfully supportive husband and family and friends who have stuck by me. I have found people to be unbelievably kind. To me, they are the heroes. I think of my mother often and was so awed by the way she handled her cancer. She never complained so I promised myself I would do the same.

It's not that I don't have bad days, but I am so lucky and blessed. Having cancer and going through Katrina makes me feel like I have a secret and it's a good one. I know the true meaning of life. I know what it's like to face death square in the face. I know what it's like one minute to have a house and the next minute to have nothing. But at the same time, I've never be happier. Life becomes more precious. I think back on the time right after Katrina when we had no possessions to worry about. We got down to the bare minimum, and it's just you, God and your family. That's all that matters.

CHAPTER 15

For the love of Andrew

Patty Mele

Age 47
Stage IV breast cancer
Diagnosed 2007
Boston, Massachusetts

Overcoming challenges has always been a way of life for me. I've had multiple sclerosis (MS) since I was in college. I'm very mobile and do quite well with it. My son Andrew has a genetic metabolic disease. The easiest way to explain it is his body doesn't make enough power, like a car running out of gas. Andrew leads a very normal life and is a bright, active teenager. But without me, he doesn't tick.

In 2007, my life was very busy taking care of Andrew. Luckily, I made time to get a routine mammogram. My maternal grandmother had breast cancer, so there was a family history.

I received a call after my mammogram, telling me I needed to go back to have it retaken. After that, the doctor immediately did a biopsy and told me I had cancer in my right breast.

They did a lot of testing and determined the cancer cells were aggressive and hormone based. The lump was about five centimeters. Since I'm small-breasted, it took up my entire breast from nipple to chest wall. I never knew the lump existed because I never did breast self-exams.

But the news got even worse. After more tests, they discovered cancer had spread to my lymph nodes, liver, and lung. All of this happened rapidly, and I was in absolute shock.

It was the absolute worse feeling. I was terrified I might not be there for Andrew, and I'm sure he was, too. He was fourteen and still needed me. I've always been his lifeline and his advocate. I have done absolutely everything I could to support him. I wondered, "Will I be there when he graduates from high school?"

Because of my MS, I was accustomed to wading through medical jargon to research different treatments. I immediately began educating myself about breast cancer. I checked out books and resources on the Web to determine how I could save my life and still preserve my breast. The more I read, the more frightened I became.

I asked my doctor if I was going to die. She told me, "We're going to do everything we can to save you and beat this."

I did everything I could, too. I fought so I could be there for Andrew. I felt horrible; it wasn't fair to my son. As a teenager, I had lost both my parents within two years of each other, and I didn't want that happening to him.

I was so mad at this cancer; it was not taking me! I thought, "This can't fall apart. If he lost me, it would change the whole outcome of his life. Who was going to help Andrew reach his goals?"

Perseverance kicks in when you have a goal. I was determined to beat cancer and be there for my child. So I had this attitude that we'll get it done and get through it.

My doctor put me on a very strong chemo regimen, and I became very ill with every side effect you could imagine. I believe the MS brought on these complications. My eyesight was off, so I was afraid to drive. I developed hand, foot, and mouth disease and irritable bowl syndrome. The chronic fatigue I already had from MS became worse.

The chemo worked, however, shrinking the tumor immensely after a few months. At that point, they said they could do a lumpectomy and remove some lymph nodes.

Because that first lumpectomy did not have clear margins, my surgeon had to operate again. After sending more samples to pathology, they found there was still cancer in the lymph nodes and in my blood vessels. I went back to chemo; then had two months of daily radiation.

I think Andrew was a little angry and scared during this time. Mom had always been there and cleared the path for him; then suddenly, he couldn't depend on Mom. I remember driving him to baseball games and stopping to throw up on the side of the road.

But I realized I had to take care of myself if I was going to make it. One of the best things I did was to get help with driving my son back and forth to school. He goes to a small, private school in Providence, Rhode Island. It took me forty-five to fifty minutes each way to drive him to school. Then I had to travel forty minutes to an hour and half to Boston for treatment. To make things easier, he stayed in Rhode Island with friends a lot during that period.

I also sought help through various organizations. At my oncologist's office, I found a brochure about Hope in Bloom. I love gardening and flowers, so I called the founder and told her about my situation. Hope in Bloom came out with my local garden club and planted a gorgeous perennial garden for me. The colors were so beautiful and gave me something to look at during my chemo treatments when I was so sick. It brought color into my life, and I still love it.

Another organization that helped me was the Ellie Fund, which provided meals and housecleaning. It was absolutely wonderful! It felt uplifting to have some support because I didn't have a mother to stay and take care of me.

I started to focus on what made me happy, but had neglected because I was so busy with my son. This included reading, praying, and reconnecting with old friends. My girlfriends were so supportive. They came with me for all of my treatments and procedures and helped me with anything I needed. And they kept me laughing. That was the most important thing for me.

For instance, when I was first diagnosed, I was talking on the phone with my good friend Barbara. She mentioned a commercial that showed an advertisement on the back of a man's bald head. "I figured out what we can do," she said. "We can make money by putting an advertisement on your head when you go bald!"

I was hit a curve ball when the cancer came back two months after I was done with chemo. I thought I'd be able to wrap treatment up by my son's sophomore year; then I had to start it all over again. Two months of radiation followed. But by March 2009, all my scans and other tests were clean. To this day, they continue to show no evidence of disease.

Facing death has helped me slow down. I finally put the brakes on and took a real good look at my life. Now I try to put myself first instead of just tending to my son's and every one else's needs. I'm not as much of a people pleaser as I was prior to my diagnosis, and am rediscovering what brings happiness to my life.

I've wanted a pug dog since my son was ten years old. This spring I'm going to get one! And a bunch of my girlfriends are talking about going to Vegas to celebrate our fiftieth birthdays together.

My philosophy is to enjoy life day to day and take it from there. Once my son makes his college transition, I'll have even more time for me. For now, I want to spend next year and a half focusing on getting Andrew through high school, while still making time for myself.

I just talked with my aunt about going to Ocean City together. I love the beach, but my son wants nothing to do with it. So I told my husband, "You drive Andrew to baseball this summer; I'm going to the beach with my books and my girlfriends. I need the vitamin D!" I wouldn't have done that prior to my diagnosis.

Hope in Bloom: www.hopeinbloom.org
Ellie Fund: www.elliefund.org

CHAPTER 16

Calling all angels

Jonny Imerman

Age 34
Stage IV testicular cancer
Diagnosed 2002
Chicago, Illinois

I was twenty-six, working in commercial real estate and studying for an MBA. I went to the gym all the time and felt great. Cancer was the last thing I was thinking about. One day I suddenly doubled over in pain from the left testicle.

The ER doctor thought it was an infection and gave me penicillin. But two weeks later, it hadn't gone away. I visited a specialist who found a tumor right away. I went right into surgery to remove the testicle. The cancer had spread up into my pelvis and stomach. They told me, "This is a curable cancer, but it's mildly advanced, and we need to jump on it right away. We're going to skip radiation and go right into chemo." So I immediately started five months of chemotherapy.

It happened so fast, it was hard to understand what was going on in the beginning. I was confident, but at the same time, I prayed every morning and night and said, "If I live through this, I'll give back and find a way to improve the cancer world." It motivated me a lot just knowing that after I got my life back, I was going to do something to change things.

I was clear for about a year until a CT scan showed I had four tumors in the lymph nodes next to my spine. They performed a risky surgery in which they moved all the organs out of the way, removed the tumors, and put the organs back in. I had an eleven-inch incision with about eighty staples. I didn't know the risks at the time. Later I spoke with surgeons who told me they would never do that surgery because it's so complicated and could have left me paralyzed. Fortunately I had a great surgeon who had the experience to get the job done. I've been clear of cancer ever since. I get checkups every six months and will do that for the rest of my life.

I'm very lucky. My family's so warm, and my mom was with me every minute. My brothers flew in from all over the country to be with me during my surgeries and first chemo day. I was surrounded by love. Yet when I went to chemo, I saw so many people who were all by themselves. They looked terrified and depressed.

At the same time, I couldn't find anybody my age to connect with. I definitely had fertility and sexual concerns I didn't want to discuss with my mom, like, "Can you have children; does it hurt when you have sex?"

I banked sperm right before chemo. Ironically, a couple of years later I discovered I could have kids. I told my mom, "Since I can have kids, I'm not going to pay the $300 to keep my sperm frozen. Right away she said, "Absolutely not! If we have to, we'll pay for it. Let's just be safe!"

I'm an optimist. I figured I had beat cancer, and in two weeks I'd be back in the gym. But my body had been through the wringer, and it took me more than a year to get stronger. When I tried to get to the gym right away, I couldn't do it. I tried to lift weights and had shooting pains in my stomach. It was difficult. My friends were playing basketball, going to the gym, and going out. I was going to bed at 8 P.M. and was always tired. I couldn't do all the things I loved.

One day I went to my mom's house crying, saying, "Mom, I'm ruined. I can't play basketball anymore. I'll never be an athlete again. I'm tired and frustrated all the time." I had expected life to be easy afterwards, and it wasn't.

I wanted so badly to find another guy in his twenties who could say, "Look buddy, I get it—because I've done it. Here's how to navigate this trial." But I didn't know anyone. My friends or family couldn't do that for me. It would have inspired and motivated me to know I wasn't the first guy in the world to have this.

After I was done with treatment, I went online to find somebody with testicular cancer so I could be that "big brother" I never had. I couldn't find him. I thought, "If I can't find a guy to help, how are they ever going to find me?" I realized a lot of people felt like I did—like "I'm the only one going through it."

Most people don't have that kind of support network. That was one of the reasons I created Imerman Angels. I started recruiting long-term survivors to mentor other survivors, doing it on a part-time basis while working in my real estate job. In the beginning, I didn't want to focus on fundraising because I'd have to spend all my spare time on that. When people started making donations, I said, "We're not even a 501(c)3; I don't want to deal with the paperwork. I just want to motivate and connect with people."

It wasn't until the summer of 2006 when I finally looked at my whole life and said to myself, "This is my life's mission; this is what I want to do full-time." I opened a bank account and started accepting donations. It was just me that first year. Then I started hiring employees.

Now we have five full-time employees and more than two thousand survivors in our worldwide network. We get really fired up; we want to do so much more. People try to brave it alone when they don't have to because there are so many survivors out there who want to give back and inspire others. They have already been down the same road and are coming back to the starting line to help others get to the finish.

We have a unique funding strategy. The most aggressive thing we do is send an email invitation to an event. All the donations come unsolicited, usually from someone who's been helped by us, or from their family and friends. It's all organic; I call it the gratitude model. We just focus on our purpose, and everything else works out.

It's important to get those positive stories out there. There's a Lance Armstrong for every cancer, someone whose doctor said, "You're not going to make it. You have maybe six months to a year." Then years later, the person is doing great. Our job is to get that Lance Armstrong hooked up with someone who has the same disease, and say "Here's a guy who did it; you can do it, too."

There is such a need out there for connection. Our five-year goal is to have a match for everyone within twenty-four hours who is the same age, gender, and cancer. So no one fights without knowing a survivor.

Cancer is a unique experience, especially for young people and those with rare cancers. I think there's an instant bond between cancer survivors. When I meet another survivor, I feel like I already know the person. We both get it. When you drill down and match people who are the same age and have the same cancer and treatments, then you get an even stronger connection.

We recently heard from a forty-year-old woman from Chicago who beat leukemia and mentored a leukemia survivor from Germany. The German woman sent her and us an email that said, "Thank you, my angels from America. Your friendship throughout the last year has meant the world to me. I'm healthy now. Now it's my turn to help someone else and give back. I want to be a mentor."

It's a beautiful thing! I love seeing when one of our angels helps somebody, especially on a global perspective. That's the cycle of giving back. It doesn't really matter where someone lives. If two people speak the same language and have the same cancer, we can make a match. We've donated calling cards so they can call each other and travel expenses so they can meet each other. It's zero cost to them; that's never going to change.

In addition to friendship and support, long-term survivors can offer valuable information. They already know about available resources and what to expect after treatment. If that information isn't shared to help another person, it's essentially wasted.

Likewise, I never want to waste an opportunity to match up survivors. I travel all over the country, going to conferences and cancer centers where I talk to nurses, doctors, and social workers. We try to get them fired up about our idea because they are the ones who talk to cancer patients.

I'm out of town 70 percent of the time spreading the word about Imerman Angels. It takes a lot of time; it's a life mission and I never turn it off. I've always been high-energy. The only difference between pre cancer and post cancer is that energy is focused now.

I do take time to play basketball with my buddies and go to the gym, but I wear an Imerman Angels T-shirt every day. I don't want to miss one opportunity when a survivor can tap me on the shoulder and ask, "Hey what's Imerman Angels?" Every time that happens, we're one step closer to helping someone who's all alone.

My travel schedule makes relationships difficult. A friend was kidding around and said, "You're only going to date another survivor because she'll get it." I think in time I'll meet the right girl, but cancer has taught me to live one day at a time. If you wake up happy and go to bed happy knowing you're helping people, you can be grateful for that. Right now my biggest focus is Imerman Angels.

I mentor a lot. I have a buddy who texted me this morning who just finished surgery for a very rare sarcoma. He's in Baltimore, and I keep in touch with him all the time. I have several guys in Chicago with different cancers and one with testicular cancer. We clicked because we're young guys. We've partnered them with other angels, but I keep in touch with them, too. I love it; one of my favorite things in the world is to be a friend to someone else and be that beacon of light.

There is no question in my mind I had cancer because I was supposed to figure out a way to make the system better. I think people go through certain things because there's a larger purpose. They see a gap and get passionate about filling it. I'm one of those guys.

I get so much enjoyment and fulfillment from my job. If I could pick one job in the world, I would have this one. There are lots of hugs and high-fives around our office. We get so excited when we match someone up. Our survivors are clearly changing people's perspectives. That's what gets us stoked and motivated: knowing we're making a difference.

Imerman Angels: www.imermanangels.org

Support

Discussion Questions

1. How did having support make a difference for the people in this book?
2. Are you comfortable asking for support? What suggestions would you give to people wondering how to support a loved one with cancer?
3. Who are the most important people in your life? How has their support helped you?
4. What have been your experiences attending support groups? Do you find them helpful? Why or why not?
5. Are you open talking to others about your situation? Why or why not?

Part IV

Perseverance

CHAPTER 17

Every day is a good day

Dave Massey

Age 51
Two-time survivor, stage IV germ cell cancer
Diagnosed 1986 and 1997
New Orleans, Louisiana

When my cancer was first discovered, my fate seemed sealed. The doctor told me if I wanted to live even six months, both my legs would need to be amputated at the hip. Thankfully, I found another doctor who disagreed. I was successfully treated with legs intact.

Eleven years later, in 1997, doctors found a tumor growing in my chest. The forecast was again a gloomy six months or less to live.

In total, I spent more than eighteen months in the hospital, completing nineteen courses of chemo, fourteen radiation treatments, and the removal of my left lung. I have no feeling in my hands and feet and have 50 percent hearing loss due to side effects from heavy doses of chemo.

Yet, at age fifty-one, I am healthier and happier than ever and recently completed my second 26.2 mile marathon in New Orleans.

I now travel the country sharing my story and what I have learned from having cancer. I feel strongly that staying active during and after treatment was vital to my survival and is one of the main reasons I thrive now. I have also learned how vital good nutrition is to surviving and being well.

Because exercise and nutrition play such an important role, I co-founded a 501(c)(3) nonprofit corporation called Surviving Well with my wife Karen, a survivor of childhood leukemia. Surviving Well promotes mental and physical health, fitness, and overall well being. While our message is useful to everyone, we give special attention to cancer survivors, their loved ones, and health care providers.

I heard another cancer survivor at one of my presentations share, "Cancer has given me permission to live the life I should." I love this because it basically sums up my whole experience.

My life seemed typical of many young men before I was first diagnosed with cancer at age twenty-nine. I was married, had a nine-month-old daughter, and worked long hours as a shop foreman at a custom furniture company. In my spare time, I was building a new house, doing most of the work myself. In hindsight, I was working too much and was over-stressed.

Everything began to change one day when I ran to catch the phone in the shop. A sudden pain struck my left hip, as though I had pulled a muscle. I tried to ignore it but I couldn't shake it, and the pain worsened.

When the pain became overwhelming, I went to a specialist who diagnosed the problem as bursitis (fluid in the joint). Two months of cortisone shots and physical therapy only made matters worse. Finally, my doctor took X-rays. My hip and legs were so eaten up with tumors, they looked like Swiss cheese.

My doctor immediately referred me to an oncologist. That's when I met "Dr. Doom and Gloom," as I call him, who wanted to chop off my legs to give me six months to live. Without the amputations, he said I would probably not make it six weeks. I kindly told him what

I thought of his plan, something to the effect of, "That sucks; I don't think so!"

I knew from day one that I wasn't going to die. It never even crossed my mind that I might not make it, even with the doctor's gloomy prediction. The doctor didn't even determine what type of cancer I had. His motto appeared to be, "When in doubt, cut it out."

I got a second opinion from Dr. Jayne Gurtler at East Jefferson General Hospital in Metairie, Louisiana. She didn't know what kind of tumors I had either, but she disagreed with my first doctor. She referred me to M.D. Anderson Cancer Center in Houston.

It took a month for the doctors there to diagnose the cancer. It was in the bone, but wasn't bone cancer. A hip biopsy showed that it was germ cell cancer. It's very rare; similar to testicular cancer. Why these tumors were in the bones of my legs is still a mystery. In twenty-three years, I've only spoken to one other person who has had this same form of cancer.

Once the diagnosis came, the doctors told me they could save my legs, but the chemo would be very harsh. At times it felt as though they would figure out how much chemo would kill me, dump a little bit out, and give me the rest. In fact, the chemo almost killed me twice. My white blood counts became so low, they had to put me in isolation.

After nine months of chemo and radiation treatments, I went home cancer-free. I went back to the same life: same job, working the same long hours, spending time with my daughter. Now there was new stress: $40,000 worth of debt. Medical bills, unpaid personal bills, and mortgage payments had stacked up during my nine months of unemployment.

Eleven years later in the middle of winter, I had a cough that wouldn't go away. One Saturday, I was up early cutting firewood and had a coughing fit. I couldn't catch my breath. I went to the emergency room, and the doctors there diagnosed me with pneumonia. They sent me home with antibiotics.

Two weeks later my cough was worse, so I went to see my family doctor. He took X-rays, and my lung looked solid white. A biopsy later showed that I had a grapefruit-sized tumor in my chest cavity that was tied up in the lung and the pericardial sac that surrounds my heart.

I went back to M.D. Anderson, again staying nine months while getting treatments. The side effects were horrible, and it really took a toll on me; my body was ravaged. I looked like an alien—skinny, pasty, and completely hairless, including my eyebrows. Most of my friends and family didn't think I was going to make it.

Staying active was a key ingredient to my survival. The first time I had cancer, the hospital staff wanted to transport me from place to place via a wheelchair. I refused. It took me a lot longer to get where I needed to go, but I was afraid that if I got into the wheelchair, I would never get out.

I walked all over the hospital with my crutches. The more I "crutched" around, the stronger I felt. It was an escape for me. As I felt better, I would get passes to leave the hospital, and I would use them to walk to the zoo or museum three miles away.

I remembered how beneficial this was, so I set a goal of walking two miles a day. I didn't always make it, but I always tried. When the heat became too much in Houston, my doctor told me I shouldn't walk outside anymore because I was losing too many precious electrolytes. I started walking in the pool. It was indoors and no electrolytes were lost.

Writing was also important to my survival. One of my nurses encouraged me to write a poem as a gift for my daughter, then eleven years old. The nurse read my poem and said, "It's not Shakespeare, but it's not bad. Try again."

I found it therapeutic and soon I was writing poems about the many experiences I had as a cancer patient. Before long, I had more than 60 poems.

By the end of my treatments, I had lost thirty-five pounds and developed severe neuropathy (nerve damage) in my hands and feet. I also experienced hearing loss and constant ringing in my ears. Having numb feet affected my balance to the point where I couldn't walk. The loss of sensation and resulting lack of coordination in my hands made simple tasks, such as feeding myself, writing, and basic self-care very difficult.

After I was finished with cancer treatment, I received intensive physical and occupational therapy three times a week for six months.

I had to relearn how to do simple things like washing my face and picking up small objects. On the day I "graduated" from therapy, I was able to jog one block with my physical therapist. It was such a great day!

My wife filed for divorce within a couple of years after my second triumph over cancer. This time, I had changed my life in every way to ensure that I didn't get cancer again. She didn't change with me, and we grew apart. It was hard for me when she left, but it was an opportunity to grow.

I met my second wife, Karen, in 2003. She was a runner and had recently completed a marathon. She challenged me to run a 10K race with her, and in 2004, I successfully completed my first 6.2 mile run.

From then on, I was hooked. Karen and I ran several races together and continued to run on a regular basis. In 2007, she decided to train for another marathon. I decided not to train for the marathon myself. Having only one lung was a major limitation in training for that kind of distance.

Or so I thought. In order to support her, I would tag along with Karen on her long runs. I could bow out at any time when I got tired. As she progressed, I found that I progressed, as well. Before I realized it, I completed eighteen miles with her while I was just "tagging along." I went to my doctor and got clearance from him to train for and run my own marathon. I successfully completed my first marathon in February of 2007.

Sometimes when I am on mile 20 of a long run or a marathon, I think back to the day I was released from physical therapy. It gives me the strength I need to finish.

Another milestone that year was the publication of my book, *A Good Day Anyway, My Poetic Journal of Cancer Survival*. For years, I carried the poems I wrote while in the hospital, giving copies to anyone who needed a little inspiration. So I decided to compile them into a book. Through Surviving Well, I am able to give away free copies to cancer survivors and their loved ones when I speak at cancer centers.

Today, I go to the gym two or three times a week and run on a regular basis. Every day I eat six small nutritious meals to keep my body nourished. I eat like my grandmother used to cook—using fresh, whole food.

I no longer work and stress too much. My mother often told me, "Things always work out." Mothers are usually right. As I get older, I realize she is talking about faith. My time is now spent traveling the country with Karen, talking to anyone who will listen, and building Surviving Well. We don't have a lot, but I've found the less stuff we have, the happier we are.

Once you've had cancer, everything else seems easy. It's amazing how when you change the way you look at the world, the world changes. You just have to have faith it's going to work out, and it always does.

All the good things in my life happened because of what looked like a challenge. If I could go back and change having cancer, I wouldn't... because I wouldn't be as happy as I am now.

For information about Surviving Well, contact Dave at dave@agoodday.org.

CHAPTER 18

A work of art

Yvonne Cooper

Age 57
Leiomyosarcoma
Diagnosed 2003
Cincinnati, Ohio

My father was a doctor and had high expectations of us. My two siblings became doctors, but I was the odd one. In a way, I was nurtured more because I was so different. In high school, I had a fabulous art teacher who was very supportive. That's when I found out that I like to manipulate materials. In college, I discovered that I really liked getting down and dirty in the clay.

Even though it was my degree in college, people who knew me for years didn't know I did ceramics. That's because I left a lot of myself hidden. I only showed people my roles like "Mom" and "Wife;" not the real Yvonne. I don't think *I* really knew who Yvonne was; I was too busy doing everything for everybody else.

I stopped doing ceramics to take care of the kids, going back to it from time to time. After I was diagnosed, I decided I needed to find my voice and express what was going on for me, so ceramics became a very important vehicle to me.

Perhaps my focus on others is why I didn't get immediately alarmed when I noticed my belly was growing like nobody's business. I looked like I was four to six months pregnant, but I thought it was menopause. When I pressed my belly, it felt hard. But I noticed when I hugged other women my age, they were squishier. That was my first clue. The second clue was that I developed a bowel obstruction.

I went to a doctor who was a friend. When she looked at my stomach, her eyes got as big as saucers. She scheduled a CT scan the following day, and recommended a surgeon who performed a complete hysterectomy the next week.

The tumor was thirty centimeters, very aggressive and fast-growing. The diagnosis: leiomyosarcoma (LMS), a very rare cancer of the soft tissue. Only 5 percent of cancers are sarcomas and only 1 percent are leiomyosarcomas. You can get them on the shoulder, thigh, heart, or any smooth muscle. Most women my age get them on their uterus. Mine was on my ovary, which is very unusual.

My surgeon was such a gift because he didn't give me a staging or prognosis. He never told me it was this very terrible cancer. He told my husband, but he didn't tell me. My husband said, "You don't want to know because it's really bad. We won't talk about it; we'll just deal with it." I was not immediately sucked into the thought, "I'm going to die." It was quite apparent later in the process, however, that this could really take me out.

Only a month after I completed eight grueling chemo treatments, the cancer came back like an explosion. The tumor had already grown to eight centimeters. So it was back to the operating table. My surgeon told me it was very difficult to remove because of adhesions. Again, he recommended chemotherapy. I felt inside, "I'm not listening to you guys anymore. I'm going to see what's good for me."

I decided to travel to Mexico to do a multilevel alternative approach to healing. I stayed there a month, receiving a daily regime of organic food, vitamin drips, and antioxidants. I met many other survivors, listened to them, and most important of all, listened to me. I found my voice.

I went home, continuing my treatments. Much to my dismay, I had another recurrence within three months. At that point, I told myself, "Yvonne, you better read up on this one because it doesn't seem like it's going away." After extensive research on the Internet, I found an online LMS group and began gathering information on an online resource called Association of Cancer Online Resources (ACOR). I started emailing people who were long-term survivors and asked what they were doing.

As I learned about my own case and read about others in the group, I found out my tumors were heavily hormone-driven, so I asked my oncologist to prescribe an aromatase inhibitor, which blocks the synthesis of estrogen. I started the medication; but incredibly, my tumor doubled in size. I went to my alternative doctor and she did an estrogen level test, and mine was off the charts. We were convinced that this tumor was caused by my body's inability to get rid of estrogen.

So my doctor said it was probably time to do surgery again. I went to three surgeons; all of them refused to do surgeries. One of the surgeons told me, "If I cut you open, it will regrow in the time it takes for you to recuperate."

Through my online support group, I found a treatment protocol for LMS that looked extremely promising. The Bill Peeples' Antiangiogenic Inhibitor Cocktail was developed by a man in Florida whose wife was told to "make her plans for departure" after her surgeon found multiple LMS tumors throughout her abdomen. His wife went on the protocol, and three months later all of her tumors were gone. She has been alive and well since 1996.

The protocol is based on the theory of antiangiogenesis, which targets the development of blood vessels cancer cells need to survive and grow. It recommends low dose chemo treatments for active disease, along with a cocktail of supplements, which, taken at certain levels, inhibits the growth factors tumor cells express. He also has a protocol for people who don't have active disease.

I printed the information from CancerProtocol.com and sent it to my oncologist, Dr. Elyse Lower. She said, "It won't hurt to try it, Yvonne. I'm game if you are." So I went out and bought $200 worth of supplements and just started shoveling these pills down my throat. In addition, I received a couple of low dose chemotherapy injections. In three months my tumor was gone. My oncologist was so surprised, she called me herself!

Over the next three and a half years, my tumor shrunk and re-grew five or six times. If I got tired of taking all the pills, the tumor would start growing. Most people wouldn't do it, but I'm an experimenter at heart. I played with the protocol a little too much until finally the tumor got out of hand. In 2007 I had tomotherapy, a highly targeted radiation treatment, through a University of Cincinnati radiology oncologist. The following spring, in April 2008, I went to Memorial Sloan-Kettering Cancer Center in New York City to have surgery, which included removing the tumor and zapping the area with radiation. It was an extremely difficult surgery, but it worked.

I've been clean ever since. I am so lucky to have an oncologist who has seen me through the entire process. All along, she has said, "For longevity, we want to watch your bone density." I didn't think I'd be around to worry about that. She was in it for the long haul from the start—and now, so am I!

People ask how I handled all the stress and uncertainties. I couldn't have gotten through without the therapist and healer I saw every week. My husband was an unbelievable support. I also did acupuncture and continued my daily practice of meditation, as well as participating in meditation groups. I often say, "It takes a village to keep Yvonne's body here and healthy." But perhaps my best outlet during this process has been my ceramics.

My work on myself and my work in clay are one in the same. I used to just give away my pieces as gifts, but I made so much, it started to pile up. So I began doing shows and putting my work out for sale. In 2008 at my first show, I laid a bunch of my pieces out for everyone to see. It was like I was standing there naked. A woman went up to me and said, "I feel like I know you." I replied, "You do."

I use my work to demonstrate joy, determination, and grounded-ness. My pieces are the most positive things that I could ever create. They are in bright colors and include stamped messages for inspiration. Some of the quotes are mine, and some are quotes from great thinkers. A lot of my pieces have the message, "Stop. Take a breath. Focus. Open your heart."

These messages, I believe, are relevant to everyone. It's a universal principle to survive—whether it's cancer, divorce, or loss of a child. We all have in common our struggle to survive our challenges. My friends will say, "You're so great. You've had cancer." I'll say, "You lost your husband. I'd be devastated. Look at you; you're walking around!"

My work has helped me through my ups and downs. I remember texting my therapist, saying, "I have *scanxiety*! My scans are coming up in a few weeks." She replied, "Well, what does your body say?" I said, "I can't hear my body, my mind is working overtime!"

I went down into my basement studio and started working with the clay and said to myself, "Okay, get a grip; what are you doing?" It really helped me to focus.

Ceramics has also helped me get to know me better and open up with others. I made some good friends since my diagnosis—not cancer survivors, just people I've met along the way. I'm learning how to be a friend.

I'm the only one in my group of friends who has had cancer. You don't want to be just your cancer. People will say, "How are you?" I'll reply, "I'm doing fine, and when I'm not, I'll let you know." Everybody has their fears. They are all watching me and seeing how I do. I'll tell them, "It's not so bad. You don't have to die over it anymore. Even the worst prognosis, you can get through it and you come out on the other side of it and live with it."

Association of Cancer Online Resources (ACOR): www.acor.org
Cancer Protocol.com: www.cancerprotocol.com
Yvonne Cooper's Ceramics: http://www.ceramics.cooper.jp/

CHAPTER 19

Riding the distance

Jack Gray

Age 56
Stage IV prostate cancer
Diagnosed 2004
Shelby, Ohio

Cancer has been a big part of our lives. My father and father-in-law passed away from cancer. A very close friend–I'd call her my sister in everything but blood–passed away from cancer. My wife Chris has the rarest form of a rare precancerous disease called Paget's disease for which there is no cure. She has been under constant doctor's care since 2000.

So when I was diagnosed with stage IV prostate cancer that had spread to my bladder, I knew what I was up against. I had been retired four years after working as a music teacher for thirty years and was busy with my new career as a student travel planner.

I am forever grateful to my doctor who let us know he was not going to give up on me. The doctor's words to us were, "You are too young to have prostate cancer. I'm not going to be happy giving you five years; I'd rather give you thirty."

While those words were hopeful, the road certainly was not easy. One week after surgery to remove the cancer, I started a hormone-based chemo regimen which lasted three years. The drug, Lupron, eliminates the body's ability to produce testosterone, which feeds the cancer. Later I started two months of daily radiation treatments.

I told my doctors I felt like the "poster boy" for side effects, which included everything from incontinence and impotence to extreme fatigue and depression. It seemed I had everything except breast enlargement and my voice going up three octaves. Over the years, I have had numerous surgeries to address complications associated with chemo and radiation treatments, but today I'm cancer-free.

My family, especially my wife, helped me through these rough times. Chris was and continues to be my rock. Even though she has her own illness to contend with, she has never given me any reason to doubt myself.

I also gained inspiration from other cancer survivors. They were my heroes. A young man in my community named Mason was diagnosed with a very rare form of cancer at age nine and fought it valiantly for three years before he died. He never complained and did what he could do. On days when I felt absolutely horrible, I thought, "If Mason can get through the day; I can get through the day."

Lance Armstrong was another one of my heroes. In my twenties I had been a cyclist so his story struck a chord with me. I thought if he could get through his challenges, I could too. After I had been in treatment for two years, the doctor said to me, "You're well enough now; it's time to get back into some kind of physical routine. What do you like to do?"

I told him I used to like to ride before I had kids and got busy with my career. He said, "Go get yourself a bicycle and start riding again. Just do it recreationally. Ride around the block a couple of times a day."

Well I bought a bike, but I wasn't satisfied with just riding around the block. Reading Lance Armstrong's book inspired me to get back into distance cycling and support his foundation. I participated in my first LIVESTRONG Challenge, the Lance Armstrong Foundation's signature fundraising event, at the end of my chemo treatments. It was held in the foothills of the Pocono Mountains near Philadelphia. I rode forty-six miles, which to me, seemed like 146.

The next year, I rode it again with my son and it was so much easier. I now ride one of the national LIVESTRONG Challenges every year. In the last four years, I've raised about $45,000. Last year my total was in the top 3 percent. I also host a LIVESTRONG rally here in my hometown—we're getting ready to do our third rally. These things have become my passion.

No pun intended, but my bicycle is the vehicle I use to raise awareness about cancer. I have a whole program that I bring to schools, speaking to kids in third grade and up. For the younger kids, I bring my bicycle. I arrive dressed as a cyclist because that grabs their interest immediately. I tell them, "Yes, I'm a cancer survivor, but look what I'm still doing."

Even third-graders know someone who has had cancer. I let them know it's okay to talk about it and to encourage Mom and Dad to get checkups. For older students, I'll tell girls to learn about breast self-exams and encourage boys to check themselves for testicular cancer.

I also give a presentation at churches that focuses on my spiritual journey. I'm a Christian; I've always been a believer. I share how my faith helped me gain strength, courage, and a more positive attitude.

My work gives me hope. Even ten years ago, a cancer diagnosis in many cases was a death sentence. This has changed because so many people are being diagnosed earlier. We're finding cancer in people a lot sooner than we used to and at a lot earlier stage, so we have a lot more survivors. That's happening because of awareness.

My work includes encouraging and helping other cancer survivors. The most satisfying thing is to know you've made a difference in someone's life because of your experience. When I was ill, I really didn't have anyone to talk to because everyone I knew who'd had cancer was gone. Now if I know of someone who's ill in my little community, I make it my mission to contact them and do what I can to help. I try to reassure them and provide some resources they can use.

I have a friend who is going through his second cancer. He and I have become extremely close. We call ourselves the "cancer warriors." He's there for all of my rallies and helps set up for my presentations.

When people say that cancer has changed them for the better, now I understand what they mean. It reprioritizes and reorganizes your life overnight. Things that were very important to you in the past suddenly aren't important at all. What becomes most important are your faith, family, and friends.

My wife and I never put things off anymore. No one can guarantee when I go to the doctor next month that everything is going to be fine. There's no reason to believe it's not going to be, but there's no guarantee. Every day we have together is a gift

That's why we're taking my family, including my two granddaughters, now four and six, to Disney World. They were part of the reason I fought so hard to survive. I want to be here to dance at their weddings.

Riding continues to be a big part of my life. I ride ten to twenty-five miles each day, four to five times a week, all year long. In the winter I cycle in place on a trainer indoors. It's great for my health, and it feels wonderful.

When I'm on my bike, I don't have to think about cancer. I don't have to think about getting through the next day. It's liberating. We live in a beautiful area with a lot of Amish farms. I like to ride out in the country where I feel free, uninhibited. I do a lot of thinking about myself and family—not my problems. It's a release for me.

I have a photo of Lance on my desk with a quote from him that says it all: "Pain is only temporary, quitting lasts forever." I believe God knew that my love of cycling when I was in my twenties was what I was going to need later in my life. I think there's a plan, and eventually He lets you know what that is.

CHAPTER 20

Hope, faith, and Charlie

Charlie Capodanno

Age 10
Stage IV choroid plexus carcinoma (CPC)
Diagnosed 1999
Franklin, Massachusetts
As told by his mother Deirdre Carey

Charlie, my beautiful six-month-old boy, had a lemon-sized tumor in his brain. Handing him over for surgery was one of the most excruciatingly painful and terrifying experiences I've ever had. My husband John and I whispered into Charlie's ear that we loved him and to be brave. We definitely weren't prepared for the worst. It was inconceivable that he might not survive the surgery. Then they whisked him away, leaving us to wonder if the next time we held him, he might not be alive.

It was an extensive, eight-hour procedure in which they had to remove a piece of his skull to get to the tumor, cut what they could of it, then reattach the bone and sew up.

By the grace of God he came out of it wonderfully. Just hours after the surgery, still under heavy sedation, he was trying to sit up in his bed! The swelling in his head made sitting up difficult and dangerous. One nurse said, "We never saw anything like it; this child is an absolute fighter. We had to tie him to the bed!"

But that was our Charlie. When we took him home, he'd smile and coo and kick his feet in excitement for everybody who came to visit. By the third day, he was already rolling over. He was doing so well, we were optimistic... until the day we saw the doctor, whom I nicknamed the "Grim Reaper."

Once seated in his office, the doctor told us though they removed 99 percent of the tumor from his brain, cancer had leaked into his spinal fluid.

"Mr. and Mrs. Capodanno, given that Charlie is considered to be in stage IV, there is a good chance he could succumb to his disease," the Grim Reaper said. With that, the room began to spin. I tried to concentrate on what he was saying, but I couldn't. I tried focusing on his face, his lips, anything I could, but I wasn't hearing anything. It was too unbearable. I shook my head in disbelief and allowed my brain to shut down momentarily.

As he continued to deliver the diagnosis, his words were nailing us like a spray of bullets. "We've confirmed that Charlie has choroid plexus carcinoma, known as CPC. It's a very rare and dangerous form of cancer that attacks the tissues lining the ventricles in the brain and in some cases, like Charlie's, the cerebrospinal fluid."

He coldly told us Charlie had a 0 to 20 percent chance of survival. They had never before treated a patient with CPC because only ten to twenty kids in the country are diagnosed with it each year.

If the chemo didn't work, Charlie had ten months to live. He suggested a risky clinical trial that was only given to terminal patients, as well as other treatments that promised unlikely success. He sent us home to think about our options.

Once we got over our shock, we decided to get other opinions. After all, this was our son's life, and we didn't agree with the Grim Reaper. On the advice of Charlie's pediatrician, we went to see a pediatric oncologist at the Floating Hospital for Children in Boston.

When we first met Dr. Cindy Kretschmar, we thought she looked frazzled. Our impression of her totally changed when she came right over and took Charlie out of my arms, lifted him up, and said, "What a beautiful little boy!"

Our jaws dropped. The doctor overseeing Charlie's care after surgery never once placed a hand on Charlie during the three weeks he was in the hospital. I'm a caring, warm, and fuzzy kind of person. I need to be hugged and touched, and so does my child. I was impressed with her because she treated Charlie as a human, not an experiment.

She told us, "The statistics don't look good for Charlie, but we don't believe in statistics. I could pull up some reports and they wouldn't look favorable. But every child is unique. Your child is a person, not a number on a chart. There's no reason we can't try conventional chemo and see if it works."

She prescribed an aggressive protocol for him and started chemo immediately. We spent much of our time at the hospital, and even when we weren't there, we felt like we were because our house was strewn with syringes, gauze, tape, medicine droppers, and other medical supplies. John and I struggled with giving Charlie injections and changing dressings.

Charlie's brother Jay was two at the time. He understood there would be times when Dad or I would be away taking care of Charlie at the hospital. We always made sure one of us was home with him. We always said we didn't want cancer to ruin Jay's happy childhood. It was a well-orchestrated event. Neighbors and friends cooked for us for four straight months. All of us had the goal of keeping Jay's life as normal as possible.

In total, Charlie had twenty-one months of chemo, ten surgeries, and an endless number of spinal taps and tests. Charlie threw up terribly. He was so resilient; he really didn't know any better. He learned to crawl on the hospital floor and walk attached to an IV pole. Nothing slowed him down.

Every morning at 5 A.M., Charlie and I would venture into the hallway to chat with nurses and begin what would be hours of pacing the halls. We'd greet all the cleaning people, construction workers, medical staff, and security folks. They all loved Charlie and knew him by name. "That kid's the mayor of this place," Winston, the head of maintenance, would say. The room service deliveryman always would say, "I see Charlie and forget about my own troubles. Look at him, fighting for his life, with the energy of a hundred strong men!"

I was on guard the entire time during Charlie's chemotherapy. We received good news, then found out cancer was back in the spinal fluid. It was like a roller coaster, up and down. Then around Christmas in 2001, we finally received the news for which we had so desperately prayed. Charlie had just had an MRI. The phone rang, and my heart sank when I heard Dr. Kretschmar's voice. Usually, she didn't call unless it was bad news.

"Well, the scans are already back; they're perfect and his spinal fluid looks great," she said. Best of all, she announced that Charlie was officially off treatment. I sat frozen on the couch. Finally I said to myself, "What a Christmas gift! My baby is finally off treatment!"

Chemotherapy only goes into our blood. Because of the blood brain barrier, circulating blood and cerebrospinal fluid are separated. The mystery was how the cancer was gone from spinal fluid. I believe it was divine intervention.

People asked how we pulled through. We believed in miracles and the power of prayer and held on to that one glimmer of hope. If his chances were one in a million, our thought was, there's no reason he can't be the one. We had our faith, which absolutely carried us through. And we had Charlie with his amazing resilience.

I was raised by a single mom who taught us never to go around an obstacle; you have to go straight over it. That's what we did when Charlie was diagnosed. We never allowed ourselves to say, "Why us?" when Charlie was going through treatment. Attitude is the driving force of every action you take. You can live in a world of doom and gloom or you can rise above it. I had days when I didn't want to get up from the fetal position, but I was raised with the message that you had to get up.

I think my boys have the same attitude. Charlie's ten now, but he's about the size of a five year old. The doctors don't know if it's a result of chemo or if it might have happened even if he didn't have cancer. He plays on a basketball team though, and wants to be an NBA player. He's actually an excellent player and also plays baseball and flag football. His fine motor skills are lacking but his gross motor skills are wonderful. It blows the doctors away.

When some boys called him a shrimp, he said, "It doesn't matter how tall I am; I'm a cancer survivor and I'm brave." People can't tell him he can't do things.

He loves to smile and make people laugh and has incredible dance moves. He's just a funny character. He struggles with learning and gets some special assistance in reading and math. They believe it's a result of where the tumor was removed. We know he's never going to be a straight-A student, but we don't care. We just want Charlie to be happy.

When Charlie was diagnosed, I made a promise to God that if he survived, I would do everything in my power to make people believe in miracles. We live in a cynical world; people need to be reminded that miracles happen every day. So after he was done with treatments, I started writing my book, *Hope, Faith and Charlie*. The title reflects how our hope, faith, and Charlie carried us through.

Sometimes I wonder what he's going to be when he grows up. I believe he's here for a reason. I want him to continue to be an inspiration to people, and the book is one way to accomplish that.

Every day I think about where we've been; the gifts we've been given. We had a huge party for Charlie's tenth birthday because ten holds a lot of significance for us. When he was diagnosed, they gave him a 10 percent chance of survival, ten months to live and a total of ten surgeries. We're looking forward to celebrating many more birthdays.

For more information or to purchase *Hope, Faith and Charlie*, visit http://www.hopefaithandcharlie.com.

CHAPTER 21

The power of participation

Daniel Levy

Age 50
Oligodendroglioma
Diagnosed 1991
Long Beach, California

I should've been ecstatic. A movie I produced, *Triumph of the Heart: The Ricky Bell Story,* had been picked up by CBS. After years of working very hard in the entertainment business, I was finally being rewarded for my efforts.

But something was wrong. I'd experienced severe headaches ever since junior high and was an expert at getting rid of them. I took acetaminophen and put Vicks VapoRub on my eyes. Then I'd take a shower and lie down until it went away.

I'd always had a high tolerance for pain, but it started to get really bad. I was seeing someone from San Mateo and flew up to stay with her at a very nice place in Napa Valley. But I couldn't enjoy the beautiful surroundings. While we were there, I had horrible headaches that couldn't be controlled with my usual methods. It was very disconcerting.

I became extremely paranoid about how people were viewing me. One night, we went to a friend's surprise thirtieth birthday party, and I thought everyone in the room was talking about me. I also got depressed. I recall lying in a pile of clothes that were strewn all over my living room floor and asking God, "What's my life all about? Has it been worthwhile? Have I had any positive effect on anyone?"

Since nothing I was doing to treat the headaches was working, I called my doctor. When he examined my eyes, he couldn't get a clear view of my optic nerve. He sent me to a neurologist that same day.

The neurologist immediately ordered a CT scan for the next morning. Following the scan, I waited in the reception room for a long time. Finally, someone came out and asked, "Did you drive here yourself?" When I nodded, she said, "Well, you're not driving yourself home!" Someone drove me in my car to Santa Monica Hospital, where I was admitted.

The CT scan had shown a tumor the size of a baseball in the front cerebral lobe of my brain. The neurosurgeon couldn't tell my family if it was malignant without a full excising and pathology. After a brief stay, he gave me steroids to relieve the swelling and medication for pain. I was scheduled for surgery in five days.

They told me I shouldn't be alone, so I went to stay with my grandmother Charlotte, who lived close to the hospital in a beautiful apartment. My first night, we enjoyed a brisket dinner that a good friend of hers had prepared. After eating, the last thing that I remember was vomiting. My grandmother called for an ambulance, and I was rushed to the hospital for what turned out to be emergency surgery in the "nick of time." Apparently my brain was under so much pressure that it shifted to the back of the skull. It later became a running joke that I never liked brisket.

The next thing I remember is waking up on a gurney with my whole family surrounding me. The neurosurgeon had already told my family I had a glioblastoma multiforme, which is the most aggressive and difficult to treat of all brain tumors. With an average five-year survival rate at 0 to 5 percent, it's also was the most deadly.

However, I didn't know any of that. All I knew was I was out of surgery and feeling better than I had in years. I thought my nightmare was over. Little did I know it was just beginning.

The evening my movie screened at the Directors Guild of America, I told my family to go. They didn't want to since I was still in the hospital, but I insisted. I wanted *someone* to experience my big night. Here I was lying in a hospital bed when I was supposed to be celebrating with my industry peers. Then a doctor walked in with a young intern from UCLA, who was looking at me like I was already ten feet under. I realized there was more to the story than what I'd thought. The doctor told me about my diagnosis and said he'd like me to meet another patient with the same type of tumor.

When I received a copy of my pathology report, I noticed there was no absolute consensus on what I had. One pathologist said I didn't have a glioblastoma, but rather an oligodendroglioma, a rare type of tumor that accounts for only 3 percent of all brain cancers. The final word came from the hospital's head pathologist who concluded it was a glioblastoma multiforme.

To learn more, I researched the National Cancer Institute's Physician Data Query, a constantly updated directory of all clinical trials in the U.S. and abroad. There I discovered my dismal 0 to 5 percent five-year life expectancy.

When they finally let me go home, they made it very clear I couldn't be alone. So I went back to my grandmother's apartment and started reading all kinds of books about overcoming cancer.

I always went to synagogue as a child, but had never been a very religious person. I was, however, always spiritual. The first night at my grandmother's, I woke up at 2 A.M. and went on the balcony. The view was fabulous, and it was the clearest night I can remember. Suddenly I felt a tremendous comforting force. It was so powerful; I began to tear up and had to go back inside. I will never forget that. I knew I wasn't alone.

When I found out my movie was airing on television, lots of family and friends gathered at my mother's house to watch. One of my closest friends brought a blank book, and everyone wrote about how I had affected their lives. I think this book was a way of answering my question, "God, what's my life all about?" It was an amazing night.

Before I began treatment, I met with my radiation oncologist to hear about my protocol. I was propped up like a book between bookends—my parents, who were seventeen years divorced. The doctor told us, "Since the tumor is beginning to cross over to the other hemisphere of your brain, we have ruled out implanting a radioactive isotope. I suggest we follow a method that will enable you to receive more radiation than was previously considered tolerable."

This bi-fractionated protocol required me to be radiated in the morning, going home for four to five hours, and then returning for a second dose. This was required because the normal cells have a thicker outer membrane and can withstand more radiation than the malignant cells. By delaying the second dose, healthy cells have a chance to rebound while the cancerous cells are slowly destroyed.

The doctor told us that I would receive an extremely high dose of radiation five days a week for six and a half weeks. "We are going to take you to the wall. As a result, you could become cognitively slower," he said. This worried me; I didn't want to change who I was. When I called the doctor that same evening, he explained that the likelihood of brain damage was extremely rare. So reluctantly, I agreed.

All along, I had this nagging feeling I was misdiagnosed. In an effort to make certain that I did, indeed, have a glioblastoma, I consulted with the head of primary benign brain tumors at UCLA. Given the inconclusive pathology report, he suggested I send my slides and blocks to their head pathologist. The pathologist ignored my materials and instead contacted the head pathologist at Santa Monica Hospital, where I'd originally been diagnosed. He agreed I definitely had a glioblastoma multiforme.

While I wasn't pleased that the pathologist at UCLA chose to usurp me, I finally accepted the harsh reality that I did have the worst possible kind of primary brain tumor. If I were to survive, I had to go beyond the bounds of current status quo treatment and explore any research that showed even the slightest promise.

I was extremely proactive and put this project—myself—first. I started researching clinical trials and hired a UCLA biomedicine student to help me. My family was one of the founders of the Concern Foundation, which raises money for innovative cancer research around the world. I phoned them to get information. Through my research, I looked for doctors whose names came up time and time again. I tapped into everything I could.

I discovered a clinical trial at Duke University led by Peter Berger, a renowned pathologist. He concurred with the dissenting opinion in my initial pathology reports: I did *not* have glioblastoma. Instead I had oligodendroglioma. While it was still an aggressive grade IV tumor, my prognosis was a bit brighter. The five-year survival rate was 15 to 45 percent.

To satisfy my doctors and make sure this was the correct diagnosis, I sent my pathology slides to Johns Hopkins and the Armed Forces Institute of Pathology, known then as the final word in pathology. They all concluded it was oligodendroglioma.

My medical pilgrimage led me to Dr. Nicolas Vick at Northwestern University, who was considered the guru of oligodendroglioma. He used a cocktail of chemo drugs with great success. I asked my oncologist for the same chemo combination, so that's what he gave me.

When I was done with my treatments, another doctor told me I needed to take chemo for an additional year as a mop-up for any cancer cells that might be left. But I told him I didn't want to do that. So I put myself off chemo and continued to get scans.

It is now eighteen years later, and I am still cancer-free. Doctors view me as a miracle. When I look back, there were so many times I could have died. Every time I was close to death, I was saved in the nick of time.

From my experience and from talking with other cancer survivors, I realize you must accept that you may die before you can do what's necessary to go on living. Otherwise, you may freeze and not do everything you can to beat this or any other "terminal" illness.

While I credit doctors for my care, I think my perseverance paid off—both in my career and recovery. It's what helped get my movie made and my cancer healed.

The mind has a tremendous capacity to heal. I believe the act of participating in getting well helps make that happen. For that reason,

I did a lot of visualization. For example, when I had an MRI, I closed my eyes and pretended that the loud tapping noise was a line of prison guards firing their rifles at my malignant cells. At home, I would lie in bed, close my eyes, and see those spots that appear to all of us. I would label the bright spots as *bad* and dark as *good*, staring down those bright spots until they went black. This may seem somewhat ridiculous, but I'm convinced that your thoughts and imagination cause your body to secrete the chemicals necessary to destroy disease.

It made me feel a lot better to be involved with the process. I discovered I had to be my own primary care physician. You go to the doctors for their expertise, but they are fallible. I knew I needed to make the final decision about what happens to me. I took charge of my own health and my treatment. That's why I'm here today.

Concern Foundation: www.concernfoundation.org
National Cancer Institute Physician Data Query:
    www.cancer.gov/cancertopics/pdq

CHAPTER 22

Strongest Mary

Mary Jacobson

Age 55
Adenocarcinoma
Diagnosed 1995
Stanley, Virginia

I was married to a young Marine and wanted to have a baby. I was perfectly healthy, but while he was overseas, I wanted to make sure everything was okay. So I went in for a routine pap smear at the military hospital at Camp Pendleton, where we lived. One of the military doctors told me that it was positive. I asked, "What in the heck does that mean?" I didn't get the answer I wanted, so I consulted another doctor.

I went to get a third opinion from an endocrinologist. She told me, "Sit down; you're not going anywhere. This is very serious. I've been told you've gone to other doctors and this needs to stop now."

She explained I had multiple tumors in the glandular walls of the uterus. Back then, it was so rare; they didn't have a name for it.

Now it's known as adenocarcinoma. I had maybe an 11 percent chance of surviving, she said, and needed to be treated immediately since the tumors were spreading fast.

I was devastated and didn't know what to do. I had nobody there with me. The only person I had in my life was my nine-year-old daughter Erin, so I ran home to be with her. I started crying, and she asked, "Mom, what's going on?" It was terrible to tell a child that age that Mom has a rare form of cancer and doesn't know what to do. We both started crying.

I tried to contact my husband who was out on an exercise overseas, but I couldn't reach him. I had to wait two weeks for him to call me back.

Finally, I went to a surgeon. He sat down with Erin and me and said, "The only reason they gave you an 11 percent survival rate was to give you at least a little hope. Actually, you have a 5 percent chance of surviving. When we cut you open, it's going to spread. You already have about forty tumors all over the area. If we don't do the surgery now, you're not going to make it."

He asked if they could recruit some doctors to study my case. At that point, the only similar case they knew of was a woman diagnosed in 1958. So I signed a waiver, basically signing my body over to science.

I wanted to wait, however, until I spoke to my husband. He wasn't going to come home for two months, so I scheduled the surgery for then. When I finally reached him and told him what was happening, he didn't know how to deal with the situation. He was in his twenties and didn't want to handle this crisis and raise a daughter who wasn't his. He wanted out.

The hardest part for me is that I thought you're married until death do you part. Obviously that wasn't happening. We filed for a divorce before I had the surgery.

I told the doctor, "Look, I need time to make preparations for my daughter." He said, "Mary, if you don't have the surgery, you're going to die. Let's get it done."

I had to find someone to take care of Erin. My sister had too many kids, and my mom was too old. So I asked one of my best friends to take over as a parent. She was a single lady who'd always wanted a kid and knew Erin very well. She told me, "Mary, I'll take over and make sure she has everything she needs." I felt very confident Erin would be in good hands.

I decided to buy a coffin and do a will. I had to prepare myself because the odds were that I wouldn't make it out of surgery.

When they operated, they found the cancer had eaten up some of the uterus, and the tumors were spreading all the way up to the lungs. They removed all the tumors; some of them were sent to Stanford and Princeton where three of my four doctors were studying my case.

I didn't die on the table, but I didn't wake up from the surgery either. I was in a coma for two years. Doctors and nurses at San Diego Balboa Hospital kept me alive with feeding tubes, while treating the cancer with chemo, full-body radiation, and hormones.

On the day I came out of my coma, I was lost. I just felt like I had been sleeping a bit. When the doctors came in and brought Erin into the room, I couldn't comprehend how my little girl was so much taller and more grown up.

The doctors said they had removed my uterus, part of my ovaries, and all the tumors. I was cancer-free. I was a lot heavier, too. With all the hormones they gave me, I had gained a whopping 152 pounds. I was 160 pounds when I was admitted and left weighing 302–and I was only 5 foot 4 inches tall.

While doctors were studying my case, they found fifty other women with my type of cancer. But most women had died because they didn't know how to treat it. Because of the research they performed on me, a new treatment protocol was created. Today my type of cancer is very easy to treat on an outpatient basis, and the cure rate is 80 percent. They even save the uterus so women can still have kids.

I was sent home, and one of my cousins came down and stayed a few months to help with Erin. I still had to go back to get tested every three weeks and do chemo to make sure everything was okay.

I learned that while I was in a coma, they had allowed Erin to visit. She would go to the medical school library when she couldn't stay in my room and research cancer and obesity. She was worried about me and told me, "Mom, the cancer didn't kill you, but the weight will."

Most of my family was big, so I thought maybe I was meant to be heavy. But I realized that if I didn't take care of myself now, I could die. I wanted to live to the fullest, take care of my little girl and watch her grow up.

Erin pushed me to start going to the gym every day. We called a couple of nutritionists who taught me how to eat better. I cut out fats and eliminated the massive amounts of carbohydrates I was eating. I was a sugar fanatic, and ice cream was my weakness. I learned to eat more lean meat and reduced my daily calories from 2,000 to 1,500.

When I went to the gym at the base, I saw some of my husband's old friends weightlifting. They were mad at him for walking out on me, so they decided to help me by showing me how to lift. They took over as my family and helped me take care of Erin. While I was working out, they talked with her and helped her with her homework.

This group of guys taught me lifting techniques that burned fat in different areas of my body. Because I was such a fanatic, within six months I slimmed down to 180 pounds. I started bench-pressing with a forty-five-pound bar. That felt difficult, but every day, they'd increase the weight and number of leg presses and squats.

When I began, I just wanted to lose weight; I really didn't care about getting muscular. Within a year, though, I started developing muscles. It was changing my whole outlook. The guys were really proud of me when I moved up to a 135-pound bench, so they entered me in a military competition.

I benched 148 pounds and came in second place. For my age, that was a lot to lift, so winning my first trophy was a big self-esteem builder. I was hooked. I entered a series of competitions at Camp Pendleton. By the end of it, I benched more than 200 pounds, and my body weight was down to 165 pounds.

My daughter discovered a big competition in Venice Beach and convinced me to enter. The women were more serious in this competition. I was just a rookie, but it was neat to see how many people support women in these types of events. The announcer told everyone I had just recovered from cancer, so people in the audience were cheering for me. I started to think, "Wow, I'm getting support from people who don't even know me." That gave me a bigger drive to succeed.

Over the years, I made a name for myself. One day in 2000, I met this big weightlifter at the gym who said, "I've seen your record over the years; I think you should enter the Strong Woman Competition." I said, "You have to be kidding!" He told me, "No, we've seen your numbers. You have nothing to lose."

So I went to Hawaii to compete in one of the first Strong Woman competitions. Basically the Strong Man/Woman events involve lifting boulders, 500-pound tires, and moving other large objects for speed. Out of twenty-five, I came in sixth place. That was the first of many Strong Woman competitions to come.

But I wanted to do more than win trophies. I realized I had been given a second chance and could use my abilities to help others. I had almost lost the one thing I truly loved—my little girl. No other kid should be without a mom. So I started training women who wanted to lose weight so they could be around for their kids. I'd tell them, "Once you get in the fit mode, you'll feel self-esteem and be a professional lifter in your own way." I encouraged them to set goals and get into a regimen. "Today I'm going to walk further. Tomorrow I'm going to eat better." I'd always tell them, "I helped you. Now go out and help someone else."

While I was competing, I watched Strong Men pulling trucks and thought, "I can do this if I put my mind to it. I'm going to pull a truck a whole block." That's how I came up with the idea to pull a truck for cancer research. I convinced the Ford Company to allow me to use one of their trucks. It weighed two tons, and then I added seventeen big men in the back of it—a total of 10,000 pounds. I raised $20,000, just from knocking on doors asking for donations.

I did more pulls and started attracting attention from nonprofit organizations looking for funds. In 2008 the Special Olympics contacted me asking for help. This time, I raised it to the next level by pulling a 250-ton (500,000 pounds) train. People thought it was a joke. How in the heck could I pull a train by myself? But I became the first woman to do so, and it opened a lot of doors.

One of my all-time goals was to pull a plane. So when I found out about a competition to pull an 180,000-pound Federal Express Autobus, I had to do it. I raised money from people all over the country, again donating it to the Special Olympics. This time I needed an assist from a bunch of guys, including Alex Truman and Nicolas Marts, two students from Slippery Rock University, but we were able to pull it twelve feet.

Today I hold the title as the world's Strongest Woman in my age group. Whenever I do a pull, I say, "God, you have my first step; I have the rest." That's my mission—to take that first step for people who can't. Even if I can't pull it, I'm trying with all my heart.

It's not a matter of how strong I am. I'm a normal, everyday woman. I was never athletic growing up. A lot of people look at me and say, "You don't have muscles all over the place. You don't look like a weight-lifter." I tell them we're all strong if we put our minds to it. I've heard of women who have lifted a car to save their own child.

The last words that I heard out of my daughter's mouth before I went into surgery were, "Mom, I know I might not see you again, but you're going to be the strongest mom in the world."

She gave me the title, the Strongest Mom, before anyone called me the Strongest Woman. She was crying inside, saying goodbye to her mom. I remember those words and think that's what kept me alive all that time. I'd say to myself, "I am the strongest mom, and I'm going to help other moms in the world. Hopefully something good will come out of this whole thing."

People ask me when I'm going to retire. I say, "Every year, I get stronger and better. I'm ready for the next show, ladies! This year is going to my year! I'm going overseas to defend a world title."

I've lived a rough little life and God has given me the chance to do for others. I can live to the fullest as long as I can keep my hope and love for what I'm doing. I tell other cancer survivors, "Don't be afraid there's no tomorrow. You're here today, and we're going to live to the fullest. Don't ever give up hope that you can do it."

Perseverance

Discussion Questions

1. Reading these stories, can you pinpoint times when each of the individuals could have given up, but didn't? What kept them going?
2. Can you think of an instance when you persevered through a seemingly insurmountable challenge?
3. What role do you feel perseverance plays in survival for someone with cancer?
4. Why do you think some people are more perseverant than others? Can determination be developed? How?
5. How can you tell the difference between being controlling/stubborn and perseverant/determined?

Part V

Faith

CHAPTER 23

Living to serve

Buzz Sheffield

Age 59
Stage IV carcinoid cancer
Diagnosed 2004
Cincinnati, Ohio

In April 2004, I was driving down I-75 when I suddenly doubled over from pain in my abdomen. Steering to the right, I luckily avoided an accident.

I served as a lieutenant with the Cincinnati Fire Department for thirty years before I retired, so I was used to pain and close calls. After all, I once survived falling through three stories of a burning building with nothing more than a sprained ankle. But this captured my attention. I went for a series of tests, which finally revealed the mystery.

I'll never forget. I had to be sedated for the scan, and when I woke up, my doctor looked at me with tears in his eyes. He said, "You have cancer all over your body. There is nothing we can do for you.'"

I was diagnosed with carcinoid cancer, a rare, slow moving cancer that grows anywhere in the body where hormone-producing cells exist. There were masses in my lymph nodes, liver, spine, near my abdominal aorta, and in both lobes of my lung.

The first oncologist I saw opened my chart, looked at me, closed it, and told me I had three to six months to live.

"If I were you, I'd get my affairs in order," he said. "This type of cancer you have is incurable. We can make you comfortable with pain-killers."

I was physically shaken, but I went to see another physician for a second opinion. He told me the tumors were so deep under my organs and so widespread, that I was not a candidate for surgery or chemotherapy. All they could do was to continue to monitor me and provide medication to treat my symptoms. The doctor told me my condition was very grave and seemed baffled I was doing so well.

My reaction was to turn inward and isolate myself from my friends and family. It seemed like the thing to do at the time. One day I turned on the TV and saw how many young people were dying in Iraq and Afghanistan. It helped me come out of my little pity party and remember there were others with tougher challenges than mine.

I realized I could get outside of myself by helping others, especially people around me who had cancer. Sitting at church, I heard an announcement calling for volunteers to become prayer chaplains. I signed up right away.

It's always been instinctive for me to help others, even if I had to risk my life to do it. And I always seemed to be placed in the right place at the right time. When I was ten years old, I saw a car hit a tree on my street and flip over. Without thinking, I ran up and pulled the driver and her young son out of their car. Moments later, the car exploded. I think that experience led me to become a firefighter.

But despite the danger, I always knew God had my back. When I fell three stories in that burning building, I heard a voice say, "I got you." Working for the fire department helped me face my mortality, but that voice keeps me from being afraid and encourages me to take on new challenges. It definitely has spoken to me since I was diagnosed.

That same voice speaks to me and through me as I pray with others as a chaplain. When I minister to someone who is fearful because of a cancer diagnosis, I always say, "How are you feeling right now? That's all that matters. There are so many things to be thankful for when we look around."

Myrtle Fillmore, the founder of the Unity Church, healed herself from what was then considered incurable tuberculosis. She prayed for two years, knowing that she was a child of God and her body did not inherit sickness. I tell people in similar situations they have everything they need to heal, too.

Being a chaplain gives me a sense of purpose and keeps me from feeling sorry for myself. It also reminds me of my own divinity and wholeness. I don't wake up and fear dying; I don't even think of dying. We're all going to die. I know with Spirit guiding me, I'm strong enough to survive anything. If there's a will, God always has the way. That's what motivates me to keep going.

Even when I'm in pain, I know it's serving a purpose—usually it's a reminder to slow down because I'm a very active person. I work with inner-city kids through the Boy Scouts, public schools, and neighborhood recreation centers. People thought I was crazy, but I camped out with the Scouts weeks before I had a knee replacement.

How do I do this? I deny I feel bad and center on thoughts of being whole and well. If that fails, I relax, breathe deeply, and get centered, and usually I can get rid of pain without taking medication. This allows me to function every day at a high level—and to go camping with a swollen knee.

Today, five years after my diagnosis, I bike, walk, do push-ups and sit-ups, and can swim the length of a pool without taking a breath. My oncologist tells me he's amazed at how strong I look and wishes he could bottle my spirit and give it to other patients. He just shakes his head and says, "I don't know what you're doing, but keep doing it!"

My last scans showed the cancer was stable, and months before, the spots on my lungs disappeared. If that can go away without chemo or radiation, all of it can go away; that's my mindset. One of my goals is to beat this cancer completely. What better way to lead by example than to say you were cured of a disease that you were told was incurable?

My ultimate goal, however, is to serve God by helping others. How long I'm here, it's up to Spirit. I think there is one reason why I'm doing so well: God does not want me yet.

Unity Churches: www.unity.org

CHAPTER 24

Thirty-five years and counting

Denny Seewer

Age 60
Ewing's sarcoma
Diagnosed in 1975
St. Marys, Ohio

I was twenty-five years old and employed in the production area at Goodyear in St. Marys, Ohio. Life was good. I had a reliable job, we had just bought a house, and our son, Scott, was born. My wife Theresa stayed home to raise Scott, and we were close to both our families who lived in town. We attended a Catholic church each week, and had high school friends we socialized with regularly.

Theresa and I had developed a very close relationship. We were young and had our future to look forward to. We especially appreciated our time together since we'd been separated by my tour in Vietnam from July 1971 to March 1972. In fact, I got my orders for Vietnam just two weeks before our wedding. We had already had enough character building experience for a young couple. At least that's what we thought.

I began to experience occasional pain in my left lower leg. It became so painful that I started to miss work, which was very unusual for me. I saw my family doctor several times. He prescribed muscle relaxants to dull the pain. More than once, he assured me that it was due to standing on concrete floors.

This continued into September 1975, when on yet another Sunday night I could not go to work for my 11 P.M. to 7 A.M. shift because of the aching pain in my leg. Monday morning, Theresa suggested that we go to an orthopedic specialist in nearby Lima for another opinion.

The doctor took my history and did a physical exam. He ran a small wheel with spikes up the side of my left leg, but I did not have full sensation of it. He sent me to the hospital for an X-ray. I returned to work that night.

Within days, the physician called me to say that there was an abnormal tumor in my fibula (the smaller of the two lower leg bones that supports the tibia). So a biopsy was necessary to confirm a diagnosis. I was scheduled for surgery on October 1. After my biopsy, I was sent home on crutches and told to return to the doctor's office the following week.

When Theresa and I arrived for the follow-up visit, the waiting room was empty except for the receptionist. She informed us that the doctor was home ill, but made a special trip to come in and speak to us. We felt very uncomfortable hearing this and began to assume we were not going to hear good news.

The doctor faced us from behind his desk and got right to the point. He said that I had Ewing's sarcoma, which was a malignant bone cancer most common in younger people. He offered to write a prescription for tranquilizers and suggested that I go home and enjoy my then twenty-month-old son while I could. He was sure that since I had experienced symptoms for more than eighteen months, the cancer had spread throughout my system already.

It was a surreal moment. I found myself asking how long I had to live. He indicated it wouldn't be very long due to the aggressiveness of the cancer type. We didn't know what else to ask and went through the motions of winding up our appointment. We drove home in silence and stopped to tell both of our parents and pick up Scott. Then we went home and cried—a lot.

St. Marys is a small town, and news traveled fast. We could tell that people had heard of my diagnosis simply by the way they looked at me. Oddly enough, we really wanted to talk about our situation, but everyone avoided the subject. We could go to our parents with any real needs, but most family and friends just didn't know what to say. Only one high school buddy came by occasionally and stayed in touch with me while I was home.

Again, our parents were our biggest asset. They helped with Scott and provided financial support. Money was tight since we had a limited income from sick pay and Social Security, but we always hated to accept monetary gifts from them. We made new friends, and the greatest help of all was the knowledge that people prayed for us.

I began taking radiation treatments in Lima each day in an effort to shrink the tumor. It was the beginning of what was to be a thirteen-month medical leave from work. I couldn't return to work after my surgery due to the physical demands of my job. Each day, the three of us had time to enjoy being together, but we were not optimistic.

Then one day an acquaintance called me unexpectedly. Bill Mackenbach was a very successful insurance broker in Columbus, who graduated from my high school and frequently visited St. Marys to stay at his home on the lake.

Bill had heard about my cancer and the prognosis. He was thoughtful enough to call and recommend that I get another opinion with a new, top-notch oncologist in Columbus. We were emotionally drained and not eager to set out into unfamiliar territory. But Bill was an excellent salesman and very persuasive. So we decided to pursue another physician. After all, we had nothing to lose.

When we contacted the Lima doctor about our plan, he very clearly told us that he was insulted by our considering another opinion. He even threatened to "lose complete interest in my case" if we were to go outside his care. We were intimidated enough to withdraw our question, and asked him to remain my attending physician.

Finally after talking it over with our families, we somehow garnered enough courage to call back and ask him to release copies of my records for the Columbus consult. We met with the oncologist, Dr. Warren Wheeler, who recommended a total body scan to determine if any cancer had spread. He agreed with our doctor's opinion that after eighteen months of symptoms, it was highly likely. But, miraculously, the scans showed it hadn't.

Dr. Wheeler recommended removing the fibula entirely, so I underwent a second surgery. He explained that the top half of the fibula would never be missed, but that I would have to give up running and contact sports with only the tibia supporting me.

At that time, a young man in the famous Kennedy family, who had the same diagnosis as mine, had his lower leg amputated. It seemed to us that if the Kennedys chose this option, it must be the best. But Dr. Carl Coleman, our surgeon, would not perform the amputation because he said the outcomes were no better than just removing the bone. At the time we were disappointed, but today I'm grateful to have my legs intact. Both doctors highly recommended that I enjoy Thanksgiving that year because chemotherapy would begin on December 1.

I had chemo five days straight with three weeks off in-between. They suggested we stay in a hotel the first night because I would be violently ill. After that first series, we drove two hours each way to Columbus for every treatment. I drove up, but my wife had to drive home because I was vomiting all the way. The vomiting continued into the night, and then we would get up and do it again the next day. Fortunately, our son was enjoying time with grandparents on these dedicated weeks.

The chemo took me down to 135 pounds; I was looking pretty lifeless. They used high doses of drugs because I was young and, back then, it was required to arrest the cancer. I took the off-treatment weeks to eat healthy foods and build myself up again. This went on from December through July 1976.

Toward the end of treatments, I began to vomit just driving to the office for the next chemo. The smell of the place made me nauseous. Everyone in the waiting room looked like I did—emaciated.

There were times when I felt totally alone. Even my wife could not truly understand how I felt since I was the one with cancer. I didn't understand why it happened to *me*. Most days I doubted that I would ever survive.

I came to understand why it's said that if you have your health, you have everything. I felt I'd gotten through many tough times already, but they paled in comparison with the bleak outlook we had now.

I remember a turning point...but it was not a pleasant one. I felt so utterly ill from treatments, I didn't know if I wanted to live any longer. I was sitting on the toilet and vomiting into a bucket at the same time when I specifically asked God to either heal me or take me home. I had had enough, though I knew I couldn't stop the treatments.

But I did survive! My Columbus visits evolved into semiannual checkups. Every bone scan came back clean. Each chest tomography was clear from metastatic lesions. We began to get cautiously optimistic. I returned to work again in November 1976, and normal life was more than welcome.

During those five years of checkups with Dr. Wheeler, we would ask him about having more children someday. No one had ever thought of sperm banks back then to prepare for the aftereffects of chemotherapy. The urologists did several tests, and said it was a very remote chance that I could ever father children again because of the effects on my sperm count. We saw a geneticist to learn about chemotherapy's effect on potential offspring. But it was too early in the chemotherapy program to have enough statistics to give us any hope.

Basically, we were told we would not have any more children. But to Dr. Wheeler's surprise, my wife was seven months pregnant on what turned out to be my last appointment with him in July 1980. He had no answers, so he only said, "Well, I see that everything is working!"

He elaborated, saying that he (a self-proclaimed atheist) had no explanation as to why I was still alive. He did not attribute it to the surgery, radiation, chemotherapy, or any other conventional treatments. He admitted that it was beyond him. We knew it was a healing miracle from God.

I really wasn't ready to let go of my medical provider because he made me feel safe with my remission. I knew who my Great Physician was, but I had developed a lifeline here on earth that I was nervous about letting go. Even after I was released from my oncologist's care, every ache or pain caused me to suspect a recurrence. Cancer causes paranoia.

Our worries also were just starting about the potential health effects the chemotherapy might pass along to our soon-to-be-born baby boy, Aaron. Yet we were blessed that he was born healthy. Then, in 1983, we welcomed our daughter Julie to our family. What a wonderful world we had!

I now get annual physicals with all the related tests to keep tabs on my health. My internist continues to ask me questions about my history. I think it's because he also does not understand how I can be cancer-free at this point. But all my tests have had good results.

It's been nearly thirty-five years since I battled cancer. I don't think any family goes through this and says life is the same as it was before cancer. I appreciate life, and each day is good. We are satisfied with the little things. Physically I feel very good, but barely a week goes by when my experiences don't resurface in my mind.

It is extremely hard when we hear of someone else who has been told that they have cancer. Over the years, we've received numerous contacts from people who want to know if I'll talk with their family or acquaintance and share my experience. Everyone hears of the cases that are terminal, but not enough is relayed about survivors. We feel God has comforted us so we can be a comfort to others.

Theresa is my best friend and inspiration. With all we have been through, she has always been there for me. Words cannot define my admiration for her ability to hold the family together, as a young mother at age twenty-four, during such a challenging time.

Theresa and I firmly believe that God not only healed me, but has blessed us and carried us to where we are today. We know that He still carries us every day. We have three healthy children, two lovely daughters-in-law, and two grandsons Mitchell and Morgan (better know as M&M)—the "dessert of our lives."

My advice to anyone facing a grim cancer diagnosis is to please never give up. God didn't create you to go through this life and its unexpected turns all alone. The day will come when we will all get to see God face to face. It is then when we will have the opportunity to ask why. But maybe that won't matter, because His presence will reveal everything.

CHAPTER 25

Hangin' on faith

Kathy Wood

Age 43
Stage IV breast cancer
Diagnosed 1998 and 2002
Raleigh, North Carolina

Climbing a mountain led me to find my breast cancer. I think it's a good analogy for my cancer experience. This has been an uphill battle, but it has certainly brought me to a higher place with God.

In 1998, my husband Brian, two-year-old son Jarrett, and I went on vacation to visit friends in Monument, Colorado. We spent the day hiking in the mountains. Afterwards, I was sore from head to toe. I was rubbing my muscles under my arm when I felt it—a small, hard lump.

I was thirty-two, too young to get a mammogram. I never did breast self-examinations. I decided to make an appointment with my OB/Gyn to check it out when we returned.

My doctor was unconcerned at first, and said that he'd just keep an eye on it. Then he reconsidered and ordered a mammogram. So I went.

Next I was told they now needed to do a sonogram. Then I was called back to retake the mammogram. I was getting annoyed and asked to talk to the radiologist. I thought, "This is nothing. There are other things I should be doing." When the radiologist told me I needed to get a biopsy, I went from annoyance to shock.

The biopsy showed I indeed had breast cancer. When my surgeon did not get all the cancer with the first surgery, I moved to a teaching hospital for my second surgery. Still they did not get clear margins but determined twenty-two of twenty-four lymph nodes tested positive for cancer. When I learned I had multiple tumors in my right breast, I had a mastectomy.

I was very interested in the whole process and enjoyed learning about my body and God's amazing design. I reviewed all the X-rays, PET scans, and MRIs, and even asked to see my pathology slides. They took me down to the basement where they were kept. The pathologists were thrilled. They never had patients down there before.

My oncologist was aggressive—for good reason. My cancer was fast-growing, so he put me on an accelerated chemo schedule. I went every two weeks and received the hardest stuff they had back then.

But somehow we maintained a sense of humor. My sister Carolyn convinced me to cheer on the chemo. I was getting Adriamycin and Cytoxan, two particularly strong drugs known for their toxicity. We would cheer, "Go Adrian! Go Cy!" when they started administering it.

The next step the doctor recommended was to get a stem cell transplant. This involves harvesting my own stem cells, which are then radiated then injected back into my body. This was done to help encourage my body to heal after high doses of chemo were injected over a period of a few days. Making the decision to undergo this monthlong and extremely risky process was very difficult for us.

When I was in the hospital, I became very sick. They ordered food for me every day, but I couldn't eat it. The smell of it made me nauseous. It would have been hard to eat anyway since the chemo caused terrible peeling and sores in my mouth and down my throat.

My faith definitely kept me going. I felt God's protection. I had many, many people around the globe who prayed for me. One Sunday, a woman came up to me after church and asked if she could be my prayer warrior. I didn't know what that meant but I liked the sound of it. She later told me she got down on her knees and prayed for me every day.

One of the prayers that helped me when I had my stem cell transplant was that God's angels were watching over me. I can't tell you how many times I visualized that while I was in the hospital. I also had a vision of a white wall protecting my family, making sure we were cared for. I called this my "prayer wall" because I knew it came from all those people's prayers.

There was one point when I felt confused and frustrated about what God wanted me to do. Should I go to a faith healer? Should I believe He'd heal me and take no further treatment? Or should I continue down this path of chemo? Where was my prayer wall? I had a vision that it was far away, covered in vines. I felt even more confused, alone, and scared now.

I headed to church for a weekly supper, determined to find one of the ministers to speak with immediately! I found none but did run into a dear friend. She reminded me that all God wanted was for us to believe in Him and to accept the gift of forgiveness He offered through Jesus.

I immediately felt His peace again. It made no sense to feel this amazing peace during this time, but I'd felt it all along since my diagnosis. I stepped outside and saw God's hand holding a sickle clearing away the vines and weeds. I know it sounds crazy, but I saw it. And from that point on, I have never doubted Him again.

The next and final step in my treatment was radiation. I received a maximum dosage of radiation to my chest wall. After my treatments were over, I really struggled with food. I was desperately skinny, and my mom was more than happy to fatten me up. I couldn't taste anything for a while because the treatments stripped the taste buds off my tongue. But eventually I got better and put back on the weight I'd lost.

Four years later, Brian, Jarrett, and I had a long layover at the St. Louis airport. We were on our way to visit our family for the Thanksgiving holiday. To kill time, Brian and I tried out a chair massage.

When they were finishing, I noticed massive shaking in my hand and a feeling like pins and needles shooting up my arm. I said to Brian, "That's weird; it feels like I'm having a seizure." The only problem was he couldn't understand me because I was incoherent. I later concluded it was a pinched nerve. I blew it off until it happened again the next day.

I went to the doctor, who told me she'd keep an eye on it. But I knew something was wrong, so I found a new doctor who ordered tests. A sonogram ruled out that it was a stroke. The MRI showed a different story.

When I met with the neurologist, she asked me about thirty questions. I just wanted to know the MRI findings. Finally, she just blurted out, "You have two tumors in your brain." I didn't expect two. I was devastated.

With no time to waste, I met with my oncologist that evening. I think he was trying to give me some hope and excitedly told me he had one breast cancer patient with the same diagnosis as mine who lived twenty-six months. He said it with so much vigor and enthusiasm like it was such a wonderful thing! Twenty-six months? I told him I wanted to push that out a bit.

They put me on high doses of steroids and we began discussing options again. The surgery to remove one of the tumors was easily performed. But I was told surgery on the second was risky. They didn't know what it would do to critical parts of my brain. One mistake, and I could be paralyzed. I opted for Gamma Knife radiation therapy that was guided by an MRI and more targeted to avoid damaging healthy parts of the brain. The second procedure was performed after a month of daily full brain radiation.

I had many sleepless nights because of the high-dose steroids given to me during my treatments. During those long nights, I would add entries in a Web journal a friend set up for me. Soon, I found out that people from around the world were reading it, and it was getting more than a hundred hits a day.

When I finished treatments, I took a stained glass class, where I designed an image of a cross with a pink ribbon wrapped around it. I felt it represented me: a cancer survivor who had survived by "hangin' on faith." Brian had a cross pendant made using my design, and soon people encouraged me to sell them. I started a business doing just that in 2007. But I soon realized I was more interested in helping others discover that faith can help us endure life's challenges.

So in 2008 I created Hangin' on Faith, a ministry to provide hope and encouragement to people facing difficult situations of all types. Hangin' on Faith provides an online forum where people can share their stories about how they survived a life challenge by "hangin'" on their faith. We also send out newsletters that go to nearly five hundred people. The ministry is funded by sales of our pendants, which also serve as a symbol for people going through hard times.

It's been six years since my recurrence, so I've certainly outlived my oncologist's most hopeful prediction. I still have a mass in my brain, but they believe the cancer inside it is gone. I continue to have seizures, and have to take daily medications to prevent them. They are not life-threatening, so I try not to worry about it. I know worry doesn't help.

Today I have reason to be grateful. I have confidence in my marriage and husband. Brian was with me through all of it and even loves me nearly bald without a boob. Jarrett is such a blessing, too. Each year when school starts, the children are asked to talk about their families. He never mentions I had cancer. He's dealt with my cancer all of his life. To him, it's just who I am.

Above all, I'm grateful to God for clearing away the vines and the people who continue to surround me with a wall of prayer. I am truly blessed.

Hangin' on Faith: www.hanginonfaith.org.

CHAPTER 26

God talked to me twice

Jerry Starkes

Age 66
Esophageal cancer
Diagnosed 2002
Lubbock, Texas

Doctors gave me a 5.6 percent chance of surviving esophageal cancer. Therefore I'm a walking miracle in everyone's opinion. They never told me what my chances were; I read about it later. I think that was a good thing; it kept me positive.

They say there are five stages of grief: denial, anger, bargaining, depression, and acceptance. I'm not sure I ever got past the denial part. It never crossed my mind I wouldn't get through it. I'm an optimistic person who's always looked forward to the future. I guess my wife went through all the stages for me.

My first sign I had cancer was when I couldn't swallow—the food wouldn't go down. It started happening once a week, but got to the point of happening every day. I went to the doctor, who said, "We'd better get you scoped." That's how they discovered the cancer.

After our second trip to the hospital, we were feeling depressed and anxious about what was going to happen. Our next-door neighbor approached us with a book of daily devotionals she had written. Of course we thanked her, and the first thing we did when we walked into the house was open up the book to that day's date. On that page was Psalm 27:14—"Wait for, hope for, and expect God"–with a paragraph applying it to miracles. It was just what we needed.

I was raised in a Christian family and was always a churchgoer, but I'm not a religious fanatic. I believe in doing all things in moderation, *even moderation*. But I've had many experiences where I was directly in touch with the Holy Spirit.

I've always thought people who said God talked to them were a little weird. God talked to me twice, so I guess I'm a little weird. When I was in the hospital for surgery, I asked God, "Why are you keeping me alive? What's my purpose?" In a clear voice I heard, "Follow Me, I will lead," and "Don't get in a hurry." That gave me some comfort, and I needed it.

I had surgery to take out the esophagus and about a third of my stomach. They did what they call a *pull-through*, in which they bring the stomach up and connect it to the remaining esophagus. So my stomach dumps directly into the small intestine. The surgeons went in through the front of my torso and then through the back, cutting through muscle.

While I was in the hospital recovering from surgery I couldn't eat the whole time. They put in a feeding tube and fed me "liquid steak and potatoes," as the nurse called it. All in all, I was in the hospital for thirty days had two rounds of chemotherapy and six weeks of radiation. My shoulder locked down after surgery, and it took eight weeks of physical therapy to get it to move.

After I was finished with chemo, I went with fellow church orchestra members to a prayer group. The pastor laid hands on me, and I fell to my knees feeling like I was having a hot flash. I felt incredible pain. People who were there later said there was an aura of light shining around me like a spotlight. All of the people gasped and asked what it was. The pastor said it was the manifestation of the Holy Spirit. I think that was when the Holy Spirit began the healing process in me.

Meanwhile, I waited and hoped for God to answer the question, "What is my purpose?" One week short of a year after I first asked the question, I received the answer. I was sitting and pondering what God was trying to tell me. "I don't have the answer yet," I said to myself. I kept thinking how God had blessed me by bringing the right person at the right time with the right message.

Suddenly the Holy Spirit spoke to me: "I've been telling you that *you're* supposed to be at the right place at the right time with the right message for *other* people. But you won't know when you do it."

Today I'm always looking for opportunities to spread my message of hope and faith. When a customer comes into the music store where I work or I see someone on the street, I think, "This may be the person I'm witnessing to and don't even know it." So when an opportunity comes up, I try to give them a good, positive message and tell them my story.

My testimony always starts out with the question, "Have you ever noticed how God sends the right person at the right place at the right time with the right message?" It's amazing! How does He do that?

One of the things I recommend to people who are diagnosed is to get your prayer warriors in place. Our associate pastor was there during my surgery, as were people from church. People prayed for me locally, statewide, nationally, and even internationally. I had little kids praying for me. At the cancer center, my radiologist had a retired pastor who would take you in a room and pray for you. That was very important.

I hate to admit it, but I loved the attention. Some people withdraw, but I loved people coming in and praying over me. It was like getting strokes. You feel like you're being embraced.

My surgery has changed the way I treat food. I eat a lot of small meals because I fill up quickly and can't swallow large amounts. I lost fifty pounds on chemo and surgery and have since gained ten to fifteen back. I used to be a little large, so I'm at a very comfortable size and try to hold my weight at that.

Best of all, I had my eleventh scope ten days ago and received the best report I've ever had. I'm cancer-free, and we're tickled pink about that.

God talked to me twice in a year's time, and I'm thankful that during that difficult time in my life, I was actually able to hear Him. I'm still listening.

CHAPTER 27

From lucky to blessed

Nancy Hamm

Age 60
Hepatocellular carcinoma
Diagnosed 2006
Cincinnati, Ohio

I always felt lucky. Things always seemed to go my way. I had healthy, smart kids and a great job from which I was enjoying an early retirement. I always had high self-esteem and never thought there was anything I couldn't do. I assumed I'd always be attractive and healthy until I was a hundred.

So when I heard the words, "It's cancer," that was such a blow. I know this sounds cliché, but I never thought it would happen to me.

We had just returned from Manitoba, Canada, where we helped celebrate our friends' fiftieth wedding anniversary. I told my husband Clint that I felt bloated. He responded that it was probably from drinking beer on vacation.

Still, I was concerned. I had always been conscious of my health. In fact, I'd just had a complete health screening, including liver function, to determine if I was a candidate for cholesterol medication. I thought the bloating was a sign of ovarian cancer. I went in for a sonogram, but it came up negative.

The next week, I had severe abdominal pain while I was swimming. It didn't go away. That afternoon, Clint took me to the emergency room. After a series of tests that lasted until 4 A.M. they found I had spots in my lung and a mass in my abdomen. I was admitted to the hospital, and the next day they performed a liver biopsy to get more definitive results.

On my fifty-ninth birthday, my doctor called me with the diagnosis: hepatocellular carcinoma (primary liver cancer). It's amazing how your whole life changes in a second. When you hear, "liver cancer," you think death; it's terminal.

Three weeks later, I underwent a liver resection, which showed it was worse than they thought. My tumor was 8.8 centimeters, which is considered advanced. Because of the size of the mass, I was not a candidate for a liver transplant.

My oncologist didn't give me hope. "There's not much we can do for liver cancer, except pray that we got it all," he told me.

A month after the surgery, my oncologist applied to M.D. Anderson Cancer Center in Houston for a second opinion on my behalf. Our trip to Houston was very depressing. The cancer had returned in full force. I didn't respond as well to the previous resection as anticipated, which meant a death sentence, according to my doctors.

"On a bell curve, you have seven months to live," they told me. "But you're younger and healthier than most patients. You might live longer." They said there were three measurable tumors, one of which had extended into the portal vein. The Houston oncologist enrolled me in a clinical trial that had a 20 percent success rate of shrinking some liver tumors.

I started the chemotherapy the day before Thanksgiving. The next day, I fixed a family dinner thinking deep down it would be my last. I was so depressed that I couldn't stop crying. I got my affairs in order and started giving away things to my family. We were devastated. But we didn't give up hope.

I've always believed people could heal themselves if they knew how to do it. During my treatments, I spent a lot of time visualizing that my "soldiers" were attacking the cancer. I also listened to relaxation tapes, healing music, and prayed unceasingly.

Our three-year-old grandson Aiden was a huge inspiration for me. He and our son Kevin lived with us, and we took Aiden with us everywhere. I didn't want to die before he would remember me. I prayed that I would be able to continue to raise him. I knew this was my main purpose in life. If I ever felt down, I would think of Aiden holding my hand so he could go to sleep and saying, "I love you Grandma."

My husband Clint and oldest son Keith, were a tremendous support. Keith would always say, "You're not going to die; I'm not going to let you die."

Keith was constantly researching treatment options on the Internet. When we returned home from Houston, he told us about a new treatment he discovered on one of his searches. It was an internal radiation treatment called TheraSphere® available at the University of Louisville in Kentucky. The treatment is a targeted, nuclear-based technology that destroys cancer cells with only a minor impact on surrounding tissues. It seemed to be our only hope.

Unlike chemotherapy, the treatment had minimal side effects. Best of all, it helped shrink the tumors to the point that I was ready for a liver transplant. I began applying to transplant centers, but kept getting rejected. One transplant doctor actually told me, "If you have a transplant, it will just torture you and then you'll die."

At this point, my miracle began. My cousin Lollie, who lives in Florida, told me that about an Episcopal priest, Father Al Durance, who was known for his healing ministry. He was coming to Florida, so we decided to travel and attend his healing services. He anointed me twice.

I really feel our prayers were answered. When we came home to Cincinnati, I was scheduled for a CT scan and exploratory surgery to evaluate my condition. When I left for Florida, I had sixteen small spots on my liver. When I returned for my scan, they found nothing. My cancer was gone! My surgery was cancelled and my prayers were answered. I was finally a candidate for a liver transplant.

We celebrated my sixtieth birthday with an Alaskan cruise—on a much happier note than my fifty-ninth birthday. When we returned, I received my best gift ever: I was approved for a transplant at University Hospital in Cincinnati. It was only a matter of weeks until they called to tell me they had a donor.

Today, I have a new liver and a new life. I've changed a lot because of my experience. I'm not as particular about things anymore. I don't dust as often, and I'm less thrifty than I used to be.

Since I was diagnosed, Clint and I have taken our kids and grand-kids on three family vacations to Myrtle Beach and Florida, and on a cruise to Bermuda. To me, this is money well spent. I just want to be with my family as much as possible.

We're also helping support a family in Uganda. So far, we have pro-vided them with money to buy a goat, a cow, and a bicycle. Now we are building them a real house to replace the hut where seven of them cur-rently live. They send photos of the house to show how it is progressing and tell us that they continue to pray for me at their church.

I used to worry about my weight and being attractive. That's not as important anymore. Life is too short. Now, I spend more time in prayer. I had a team of saints I prayed to daily when I was in treatment. I never stopped praying.

I feel pretty confident and no longer have thoughts of not being around next year. I feel like I'm not finished here yet. I don't say, "I'm lucky" anymore. I say, "I'm blessed."

Faith

Discussion Questions

1. How did you feel having a sense of faith helped the individuals featured in this section?
2. Do you believe someone can have faith without belonging to a particular religion? Why or why not?
3. Do you believe in miracles? Why or why not?
4. How has having a sense of faith helped you? Can you give examples?
5. What spiritual practices do you use to build your sense of faith?

Resources

Many of the survivors featured in this book have benefited from and volunteered for the nonprofit cancer organizations listed below. A few of the individuals, such as Ann Fonfa, Jonny Imerman, Doug Ulman, and Kathy Wood, saw a need and founded organizations of their own. This is not meant to be a comprehensive list, but rather a starting point for your journey.

American Cancer Society
P.O. Box 22718
Oklahoma City, OK 73123-1718
1-800-ACS-2345 (or 1-866-228-4327 for TTY)
www.cancer.org
The American Cancer Society (ACS) is committed to fighting cancer through balanced programs of research, education, patient service, advocacy, and rehabilitation.

American Institute for Cancer Research
1759 R Street NW
Washington, DC 20009

800-843-8114

www.aicr.org

AICR helps people make choices that reduce their chances of developing cancer, including diet and exercise.

American Lung Association

1301 Pennsylvania Avenue NW

Washington, DC 20004

202-785-3355

www.lungusa.org

The American Lung Association's mission is to save lives by improving lung health and preventing lung disease.

American Red Cross

2025 E Street, NW

Washington, DC 20006

Donation Hotlines: 800-REDCROSS (800-733-2767) and

800-257-7575 (Español)

www.redcross.org

The American Red Cross is the nation's premier emergency response organization. In addition, it offers: community services that help the needy; support and comfort for military members and their families; the collection, processing and distribution of lifesaving blood and blood products; educational programs that promote health and safety; and international relief and development programs.

The Annie Appleseed Project

7319 Serrano Terrace

Delray Beach, FL 33446-2215

561-749-0084

annieappleseedpr@aol.com

www.annieappleseedproject.org

The Annie Appleseed Project explores evidence-based, integrative treatments and methods through its Web site and conferences.

Association of Cancer Online Resources

www.acor.org

A collection of online communities designed to provide timely and accurate cancer information.

Cancer Protocol.com

www.cancerprotocol.com

Cancer Protocol.com features peer-reviewed, published studies by well-known academic centers or research institutions.

Cancer Support Community: The Wellness Community/ Gilda's Club

919 18th Street, NW, Suite 54

Washington, DC 20006

888-93-WELL

www.cancersupportcommunity.org

Cancer Support Community provides professional programs of emotional support, education, and hope for people affected by cancer at no charge, so that no one faces cancer alone.

Cancer*Care*

275 Seventh Avenue

Floor 22

New York, NY 10001

800-813-HOPE

info@cancercare.org.

www.cancercare.org

Cancer*Care* is a national nonprofit organization that provides free, professional support services for anyone affected by cancer.

The Concern Foundation

1026 S. Robertson, Suite 300

Los Angeles, CA 90035

310-360-6100

www.concernfoundation.org

With 95 percent of net proceeds going directly to research, Concern has funded 554 researchers studying many forms of cancer, primarily in the areas of cancer genetics, cell biology, and immunology.

Hangin' on Faith

8218 Gadsen Court
Raleigh, NC 27613
919-524-6393
www.hanginonfaith.org

Founded by Kathy Wood, who is featured in this book, Hangin' on Faith provides hope and encouragement to people who are facing medical concerns, divorce, death, and other difficult situations.

Hope for Two

800-743-4471
info@hopefortwo.org
www.hopefortwo.org

Hope for Two: The Pregnant with Cancer Network is an organization dedicated to providing women diagnosed with cancer while pregnant with information, support, and hope.

Imerman Angels

400 W. Erie Street, Suite 405
Chicago, IL 60654
877-274-5529
info@imermanangels.org
www.imermanangels.org

Founded by Jonny Imerman, who is featured in this book, Imerman Angels partners a person fighting cancer with someone who has beaten the same type of cancer.

Lance Armstrong Foundation (LAF)

2201 E. Sixth Street
Austin, TX 78702
877-236-8820

For Cancer Support: 866-673-7205

www.livestrong.org

LAF unites people to fight cancer and pursue an agenda focused on prevention, access to screening and care, improved quality of life for survivors, and investment in research.

Leukemia and Lymphoma Society

1311 Mamaroneck Avenue, Suite 310

White Plains, NY 10605

800- 955-4572

www.lls.org

The Leukemia & Lymphoma Society (LLS) is the world's largest voluntary health organization dedicated to funding blood cancer research, education, and patient services.

Living Beyond Breast Cancer

354 West Lancaster Avenue, Suite 224

Haverford, PA 19041

484-708-1550 or 610-645-4567

mail@lbbc.org

www.lbbc.org

A national education and support organization dedicated to improving survivors' quality of life and helping them take an active role in their ongoing recovery or management of cancer.

Lung Cancer Alliance

888 16th Street NW, Suite 150

Washington, DC 20006

Lung Cancer Information Line: 800-298-2436 (9:00 A.M. to 5 P.M. Eastern Time)

info@lungcanceralliance.org

www.lungcanceralliance.org

The Lung Cancer Alliance is the only national nonprofit organization dedicated solely to patient support and advocacy for people living with lung cancer and those at risk for the disease.

National Bone Marrow Registry

3001 Broadway Street N.E.
Suite 100
Minneapolis, MN 55413-1753
(800) MARROW2 (800-627-7692)
www.marrow.org

The National Marrow Donor Program (NMDP) and its Be The Match Foundation^SM are nonprofit organizations dedicated to creating an opportunity for all patients to receive bone marrow or umbilical cord blood transplants.

National Breast Cancer Coalition

1101 17th Street, NW, Suite 1300
Washington, DC   20036
800-622-2838
www.stopbreastcancer.org

Since 1991, the National Breast Cancer Coalition has trained advocates to lobby at the national, state, and local levels for public policies that impact breast cancer research, diagnosis, and treatment.

National Call to Action on Cancer Prevention and Survivorship

c/o Canyon Ranch Institute
8600 E. Rockcliff Road
Tucson, AZ 85750
Phone: 520-239-8561
www.nctacancer.org

The National Call to Action calls on all sectors of society to take action and make the war on cancer a national priority. This includes improving cancer prevention, treatment, and survivorship.

National Cancer Institute

NCI Public Inquiries Office
6116 Executive Boulevard, Room 3036A
Bethesda, MD 20892-8322
800-4-CANCER (800-422-6237)
www.cancer.gov

The National Cancer Institute coordinates the National Cancer Program, which conducts and supports research, training, health information dissemination, and other programs. Its focus is on the cause, diagnosis, prevention, treatment, rehabilitation of cancer, and the continuing care of cancer patients and their families.

NCI also includes the Physician Data Query, its comprehensive cancer database. It contains summaries on a wide range of cancer topics, including a registry of 8000+ open and 19,000+ closed cancer clinical trials from around the world.

Pink Ribbon Girls

PO Box 33011
Cincinnati, OH 45233
513-207-7975
www.pinkribbongirls.org
Pink Ribbon Girls is a national online community that provides support and education to young breast cancer survivors.

The Susan G. Komen for the Cure

5005 LBJ Freeway, Suite 250
Dallas, TX 75244
877 GO KOMEN (877-465-6636)
www.komen.org
The world's largest grassroots network of breast cancer survivors and activists, working to save lives, empower people, ensure quality care for all, and energize science to find the cure for breast cancer.

The Ulman Fund for Young Adults

30 Corporate Center
10440 Little Patuxent Parkway
Suite G1
Columbia, MD 21044
Hours: Monday - Friday, 9 AM - 5 PM
888-393-FUND (3863)
info@ulmanfund.org
www.ulmancancerfund.org

Founded by Doug Ulman, now CEO and President of the Lance Armstrong Foundation, The Ulman Fund enhances lives by supporting, educating and connecting young adults and their loved ones who are affected by cancer.

World T.E.A.M. Sports

4416 Orofino Court
Castle Rock, CO 80108
303-663-2600
www.worldteamsports.org

World T.E.A.M. Sports is dedicated to creating soul-stirring opportunities for individuals of all abilities through the power of sports. It brings athletes of all cultures, with and without disabilities, together as one team to accomplish goals beyond what is thought possible.

Young Survival Coalition

61 Broadway, Suite 2235
New York, NY 10006
877-YSC-1011
www.youngsurvival.org

YSC works with survivors, caregivers; and the medical, research, advocacy, and legislative communities to increase the quality and quantity of life for women diagnosed with breast cancer ages 40 and under.

IN MASSACHUSETTES

The Ellie Fund

Julie Nations, Executive Director
475 Hillside Avenue
Needham, MA 02494
781-449-0100
julie@elliefund.org
www.elliefund.org

The Ellie Fund improves the health and welfare of women and families undergoing breast cancer treatment in Massachusetts. Its free services include transportation to medical appointments, childcare, housekeeping, groceries, and nutritious meals.

Hope in Bloom
202 Bussey Street
Dedham, MA 02026
781-381-3597
info@hopeinbloom.org
www.hopeinbloom.org
Hope in Bloom plants gardens free of charge at the homes of women and men undergoing treatment for breast cancer. The program operates throughout Massachusetts.

IN TEXAS

Lifeline Chaplaincy
1415 Southmore Boulevard
Houston, TX 77004
888-767-6363
www.lifelinechaplaincy.org
Lifeline Chaplaincy provides compassionate support to the seriously ill, their families and caregivers, and is dedicated to being an educational resource for crisis ministry.

CanCare
9575 Katy Freeway
Suite 428
Houston, TX 77024
888-461-0028
www.cancare.org
CanCare provides emotional support to those currently facing a battle with cancer.

IN OHIO

Cincinnati Dreams Come True
PO Box 4280
Cincinnati, OH 45242-0890
513-891-1941
www.cincinnatidreams.org

Cincinnati Dreams Come True serves children under the age of eighteen who live within a hundred mile radius of Cincinnati, or who are regular patients of Cincinnati Children's Hospital Medical Center.

Made in the USA
Monee, IL
15 March 2024

55140960R00125